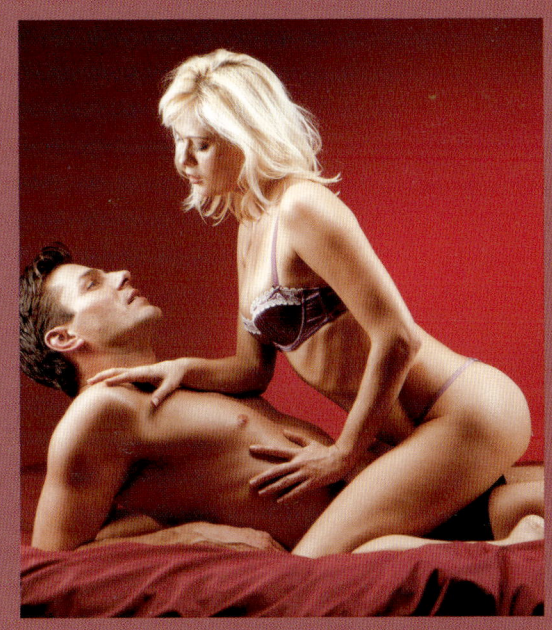

EROTIC MASSAGE

FOR LOVERS

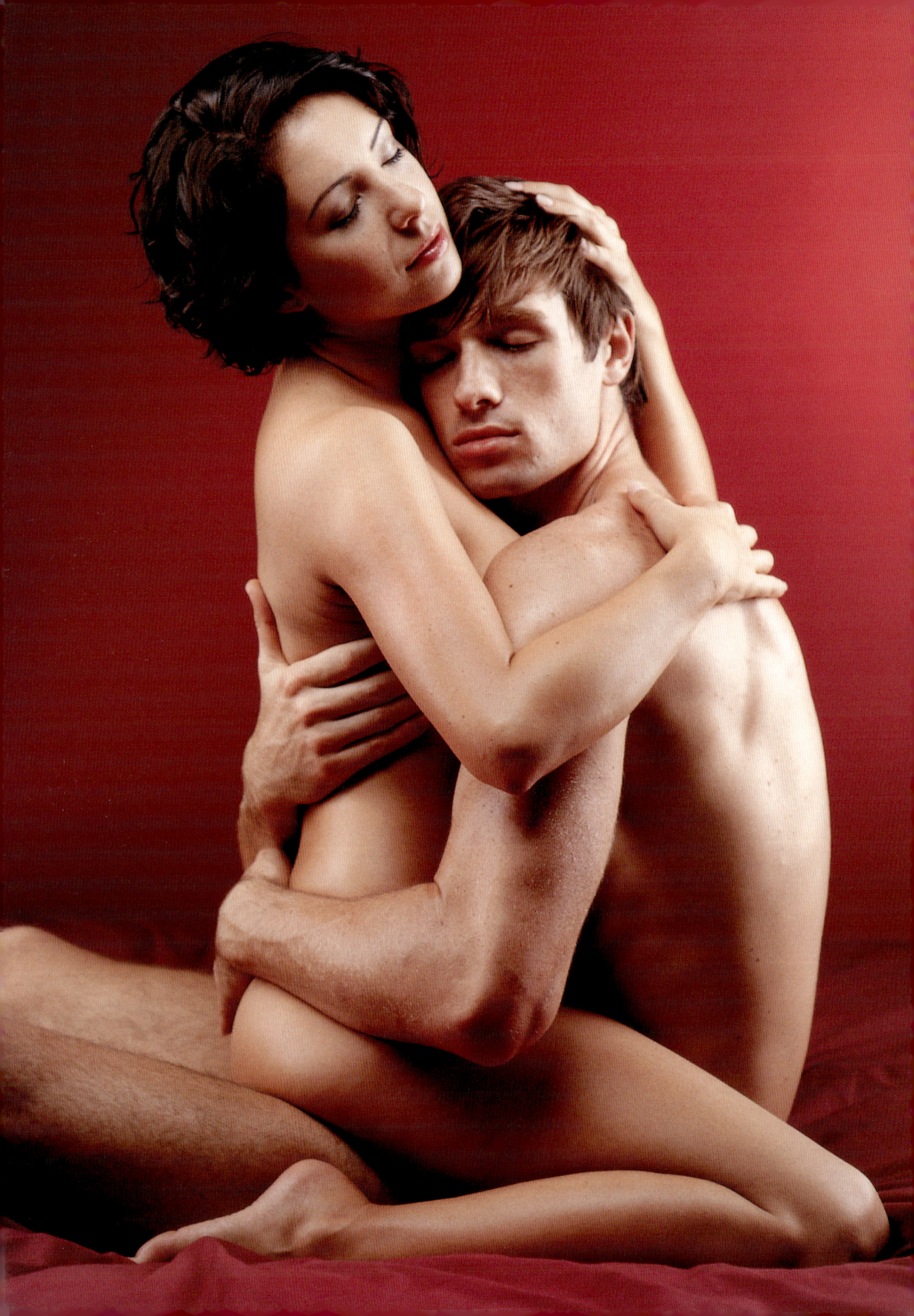

ROS WIDDOWSON & STEVE MARRIOTT

EROTIC MASSAGE

FOR LOVERS

SENSUAL TOUCH FOR INTIMACY
& ORGASMIC PLEASURE

Amorata Press

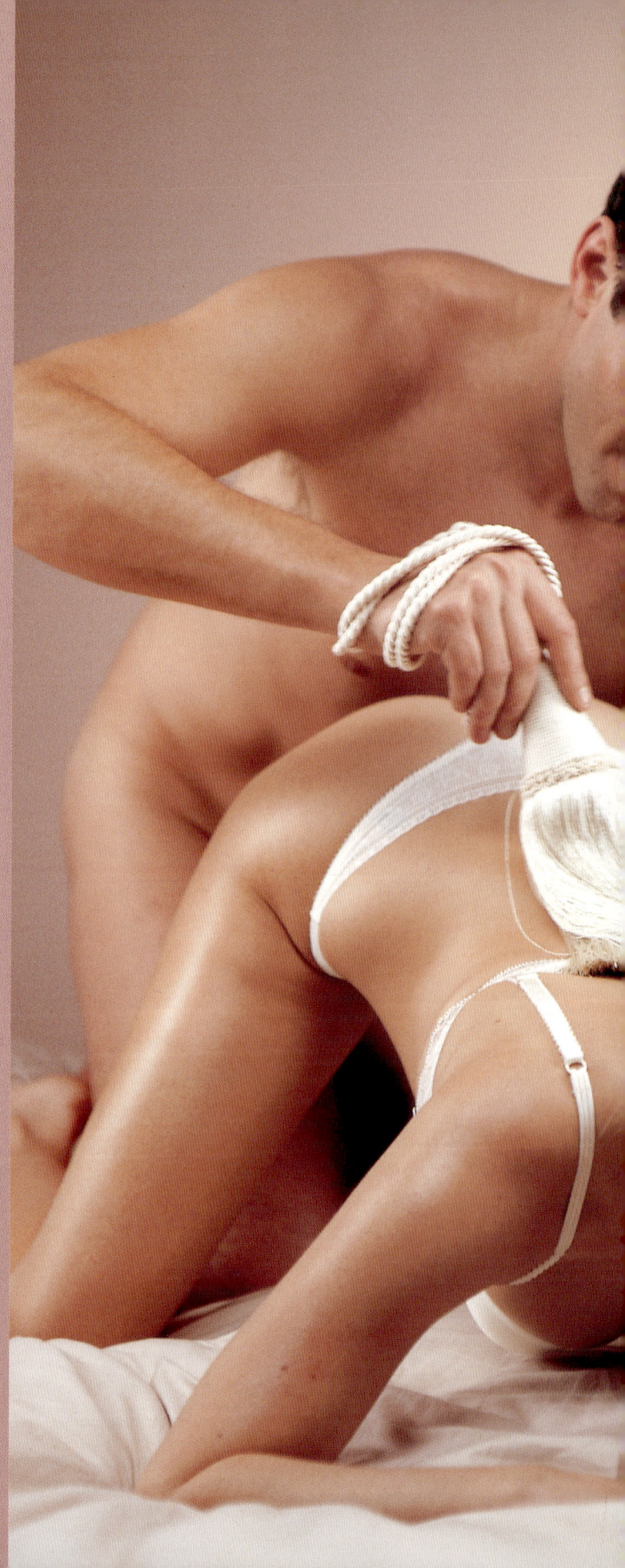

Copyright © Octopus Publishing Group 2007. All rights reserved. No part of this work may be reproduced or utilized in any form or by any means, electronic or mechanical, including photocopying, recording or by any information storage and retrieval system, without the prior written permission of the publisher.

Published in the U.S. by
AMORATA PRESS
P.O. Box 3440
Berkeley, CA 94703
www.amoratapress.com

First published as *Erotic Massage* in Great Britain in 2007 by Hamlyn, a division of Octopus Publishing Group Ltd.

ISBN10: 1-56975-612-0
ISBN13: 978-1-56975-612-6
Library of Congress Control Number 2006938827

Printed and bound in Hong Kong

10 9 8 7 6 5 4 3 2 1

Distributed by Publishers Group West

Disclaimer
Massage should not be considered a replacement for professional medical treatment: a physician should be consulted in all matters relating to health and especially in relation to any symptoms that may require diagnosis or medical attention. While the advice and information in this book are believed to be accurate, neither the author nor the publisher can accept any legal responsibility for any injury sustained while following any of the suggestions made herein.

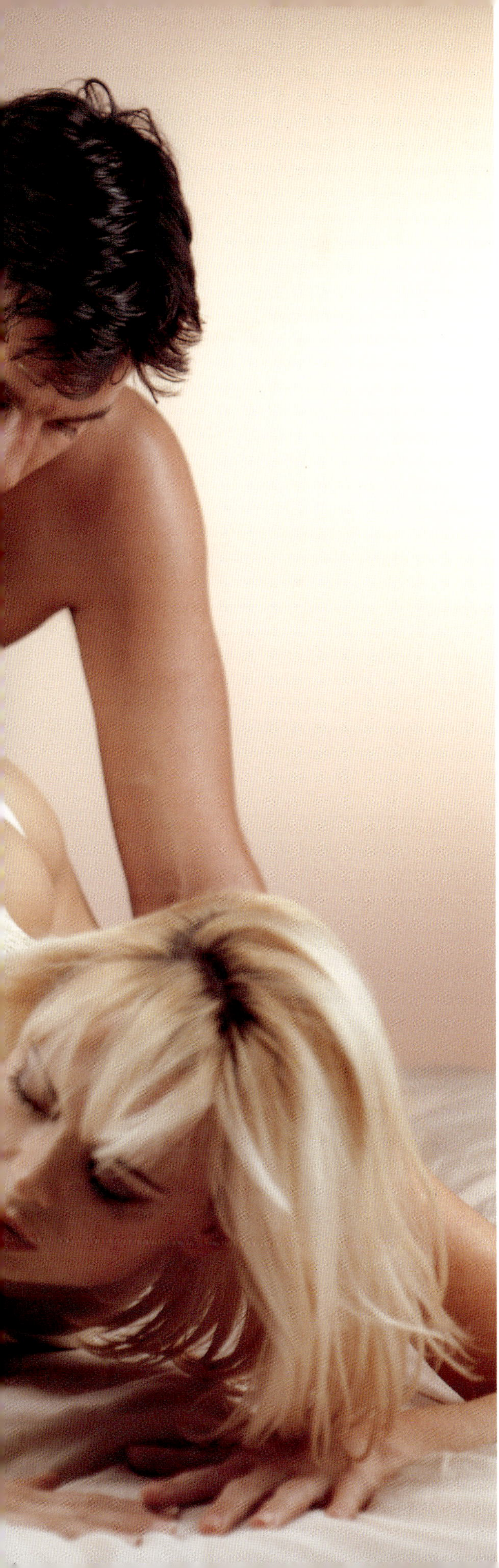

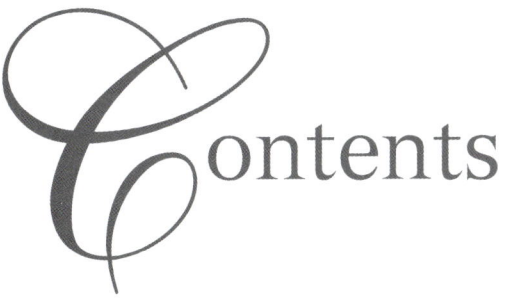
Contents

Introduction	6
Get fresh	**14**
Pleasure zones	**24**
Teasing & tantalizing	**46**
Stimulating & arousing	**58**
Beyond skin deep	**82**
Top to toe	**92**
Afterglow	**118**
Index	126
Acknowledgments	128

Introduction

Erotic massage is an exciting way to enrich an intimate relationship. It offers a subtle yet dynamic approach to communicating with someone special. An ordinary massage performs the useful functions of relaxing muscles and calming an overstretched or fatigued nervous system, but erotic massage goes far beyond this – it can be the key to another's sexual heart and sensual soul.

More than a mere sexual preliminary to lovemaking, erotic massage offers you the opportunity to profoundly deepen the intimacy between you and your partner. Whether you wish to wow a new love interest, move a relationship on to the next level after the initial honeymoon period or revitalize and renew a mature partnership, erotic massage is, at heart, a revealing process that builds trust and intimacy as it raises the temperature and expands your sexual horizons. The esoteric techniques of ancient cultures may point the way, but ecstatic union is by no means beyond the wit and capability of compassionate and ardent lovers.

Sex, and the sexual act, is not always a true expression of a lover's persona. We all wear masks to some extent and play roles where we give and take power, act outside of conditioned behavior and have quirks and inconsistencies that we may not understand ourselves. Even established couples, whether mixed or same sex, play out sex roles that do not represent their true feelings and real identity because it is easy to engage sexually on quite a superficial level. Erotic massage provides an opportunity to establish or renew sexual intimacy and a chance to explore new ground through eye contact, non-verbal communication, role play and touching with awareness. If you can do that, then even the coldest fish can learn to swim in an ocean of bliss.

Erotic massage is about taking things slowly and building mounting desire, teasing and tantalizing, stimulating and arousing, until a peak of passion leads to release. To do this successfully you must establish a physical rapport with your partner and maintain this rapport through mutual trust and communication. Eroticism is an ancient art form that can ultimately result in the sexual act of lovemaking, but it is not a prerequisite. What is, however, is patience, attention to detail, fine-tuning, rhythm, practice and performance, all of which will open up new dimensions of pleasure.

If you think the time and effort devoted to the selfless service of another is just too much bother, consider this. The gift is in the giving, yet the true rewards come back to the giver nonetheless. Lavishing attention and effort on your loved one – learning of his or her sexual landscape, likes, dislikes, passions and hang-ups – will give you a unique insight to your partner's psychology and a greater ability to pleasure him or her and, by extension, yourself.

This book can help you to learn some ways to strip away fears and insecurities, embrace acceptance, create an on-going dialogue that will expand with time and, as the energetic dance unfolds and another veil falls away, erotic stimulation and sexual passion become a gateway to paradise.

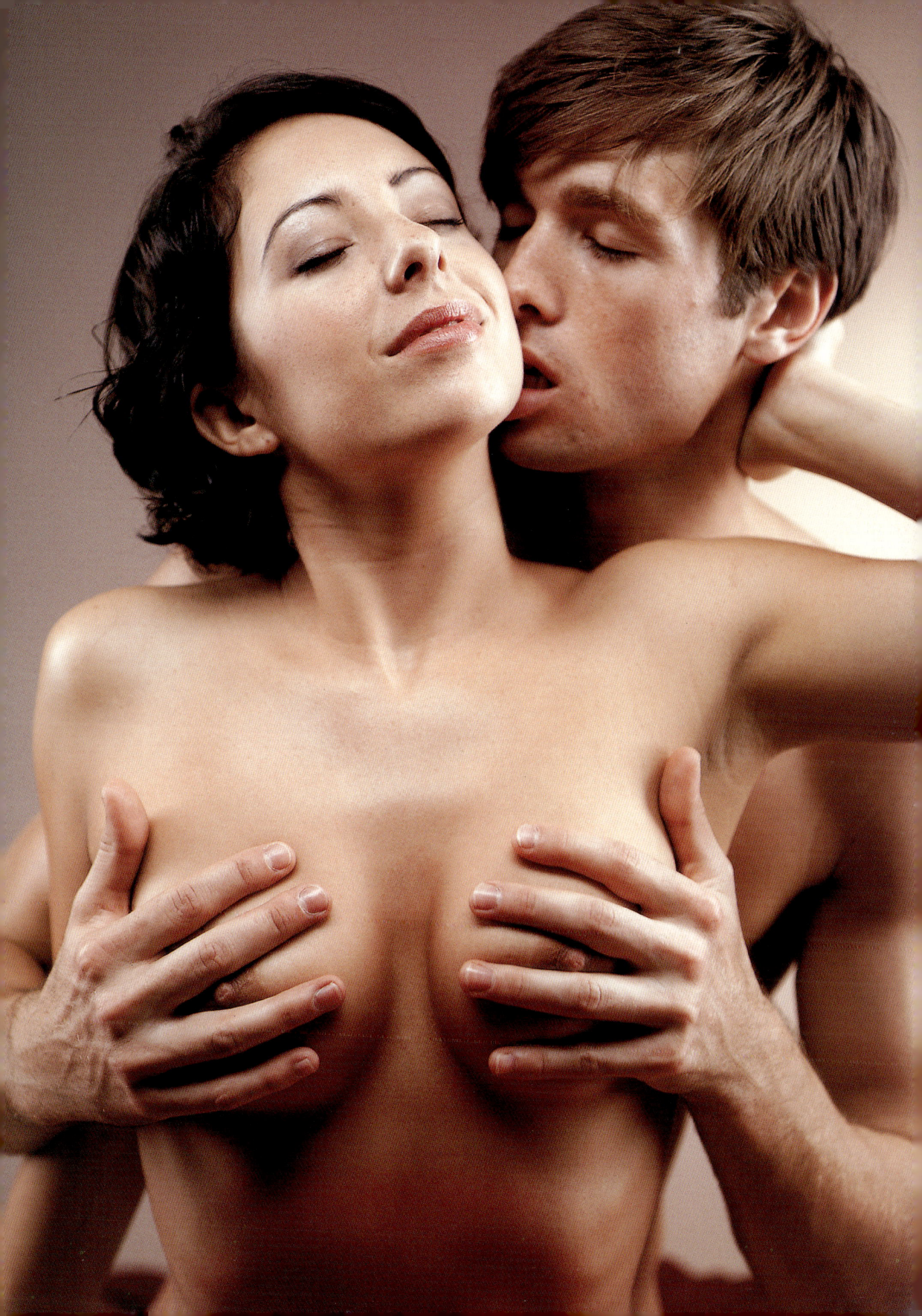

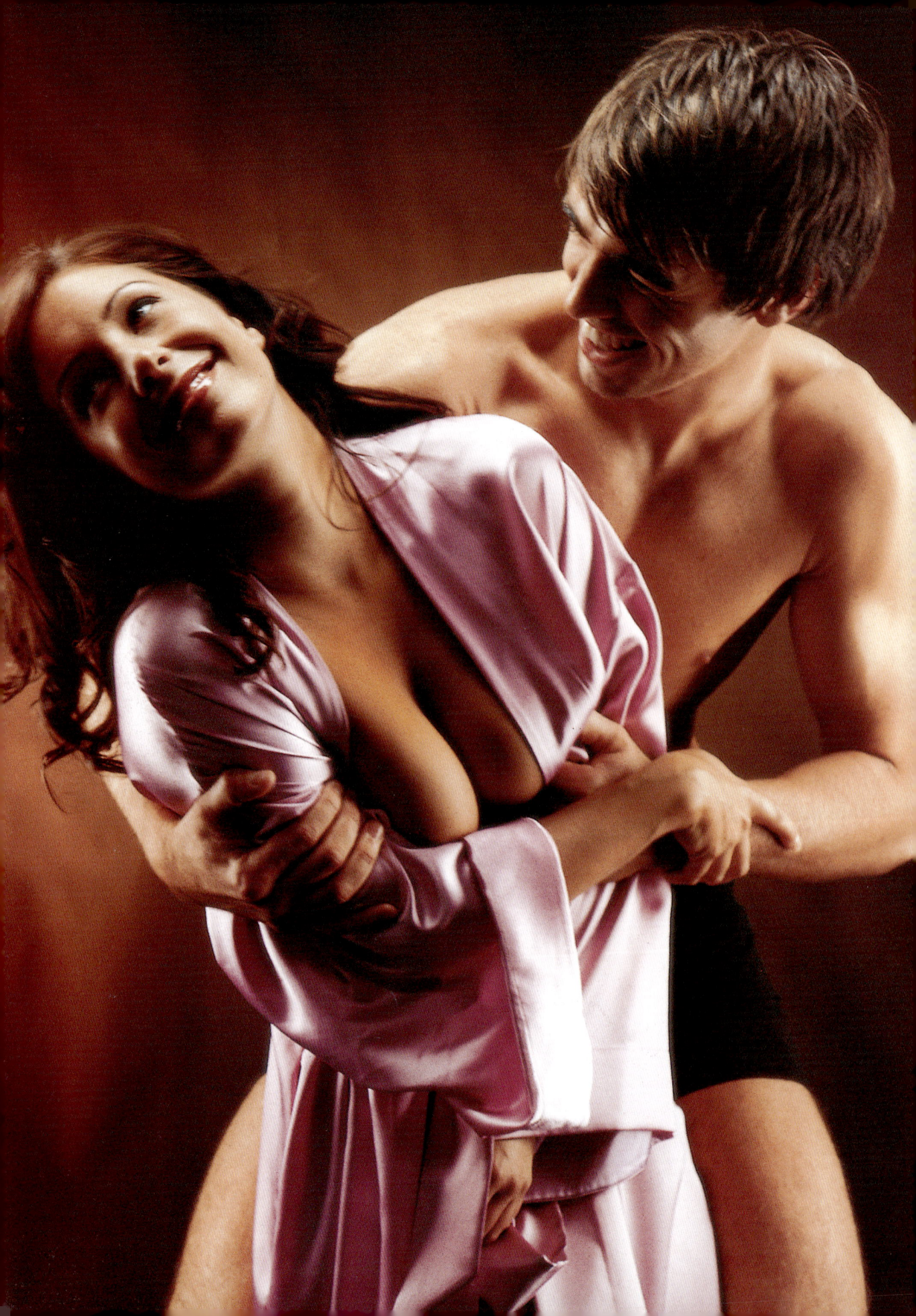

How to use this book

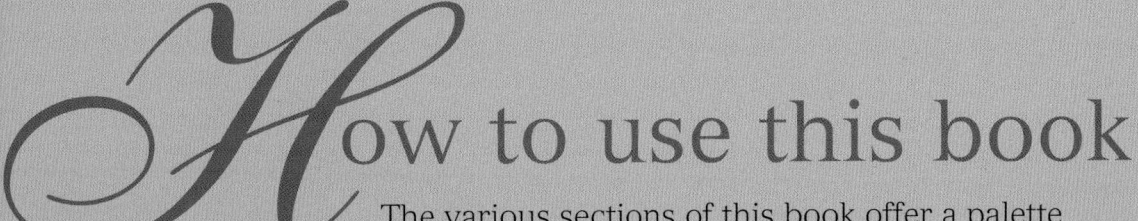

The various sections of this book offer a palette of ideas from which both you and your partner can build a repertoire of techniques. All the massages can be performed on both men and women, unless the text specifically states otherwise.

The first and last sections, *Get Fresh* (dealing with cleansing and preparing the body for erotic massage) and *Afterglow* (a leisurely and luxuriating soak) are merely suggestions rather than required stages. You might instead choose to finish your massage with a blissful and luxurious oil treatment, fun and games in the tub or champagne in bed.

If time and inclination allow, you might consider exploring *Pleasure Zones* to establish a soothing rhythm. This chapter provides a broad-ranging introduction to techniques that stimulate all the body's sensitive areas. The next chapter, *Teasing & Tantalizing* celebrates our playful natures and uses everyday objects, from feathers to basting brushes, in surprisingly novel ways!

If one or both partners are feeling sluggish or lethargic, the next chapter, *Stimulating & Arousing*, offers foundation skills that pep up and revitalize the body and lift the spirits. Designed entirely for a recipient lying face down, this sequence of strokes allows him or her to enjoy and benefit from a range of techniques without having to change position.

If one or both partners are pressed for time, you can still get ultra close and personal with *Beyond Skin Deep*, a series of statuesque Thai postures that are sculptured re-creations of classical erotic positions. These will help you to break up tension in the deep-seated muscle groups and joints and provide an arousing workout that will recharge your batteries.

The chapter *Top to Toe* outlines a complete massage sequence that starts gently and builds through medium- to deep-pressure movements and eventually travels to the more intimate areas of the body. This highly arousing sequence provides an amazing prelude to sex.

> ### "Working" and "supporting" hands
> Throughout this book reference will be made to the "working" and "supporting" hands. When you are massaging, your less dominant hand is used simply to maintain an energetic and comforting connection with your partner. Known as the "supporting" hand, it is largely static and supportive, and is used to "listen" to the reactions to your treatments. The "working" hand, whether left or right by preference, is the more active agent. The steps in the massage sequences state where you should sit in relation to your partner's body, and which hand should be used for performing each stroke. Try the stroke as suggested, but adapt your position as necessary and use your hands as you find comfortable.

a **palette** of **ideas** from which you and your partner can **build** a **repertoire** of techniques

Getting started

Before performing a single massage stroke you must prepare your massage environment. Establishing the right atmosphere and having all the essentials (and some of the luxuries) you'll need on hand allows you to proceed without interruption and maintain the erotic and pleasurable atmosphere you establish.

Your environment

In order for your massage to have the maximum benefit it is important that you pay extra special attention to the environment. Taking time and effort to set the scene and prepare for your lover makes clear your interest and kindness, and is an essential prelude to your massage. You both need to feel pampered, unhurried (ideally) and private during your erotic massage, so choose a warm, peaceful room with dim lights where you will not be disturbed. Turn off all telephones and place a "do not disturb" sign on the door, if appropriate. Music is a wonderful option, although you may miss out on the natural sounds that you both make. If the weather is warm, you might like to conduct your session outdoors in a truly natural setting. Most importantly, clear enough space – physically, emotionally and mentally – in your schedules for this special time together.

Items to have on hand

Before you begin, make sure the air in the room is fresh, but there should be no drafts. Gather together plenty of warm towels (ready for cover and comfort), water to drink (especially if you plan to drink alcohol), oils, soaps, lotions, powders and scents. If you're not using scented massage products you might like to burn an aromatherapy candle or incense that you both like. If possible use towels, robes, sheets and other fabrics made of natural materials such as cotton, silk and wool. Remove watches and jewelry.

The massage surface

Your options include using a bed, sofa, futon, outdoor chaise lounge, or the floor with blankets, towels and cushions for padding. Certain sequences, such as the Thai bodywork sequences in *Beyond Skin Deep*, can be practiced only on a solid surface with plenty of space, such as the floor. Beds can be an awkward height, but ideal if you want to fall asleep together afterward. With practice you will both learn to relax into the moves using the weight of the body to give both rhythm and depth. Don't stay static in one place – move into various positions, always working toward the heart and chest, keeping face or eye contact to pick up encouraging signs of pleasure.

Making and breaking contact

The sensitivity with which you make and break contact with your partner is of prime importance. To apply oil, talc or another massage medium, first hold your hands away from your partner's body. Pour a little of the oil into one cupped palm, then rub your palms together, including the

Avoiding the spine
Never place any pressure on the spine during massage. It is fine to massage the areas on either side of the spine, but exerting pressure directly on to the spine could cause serious damage.

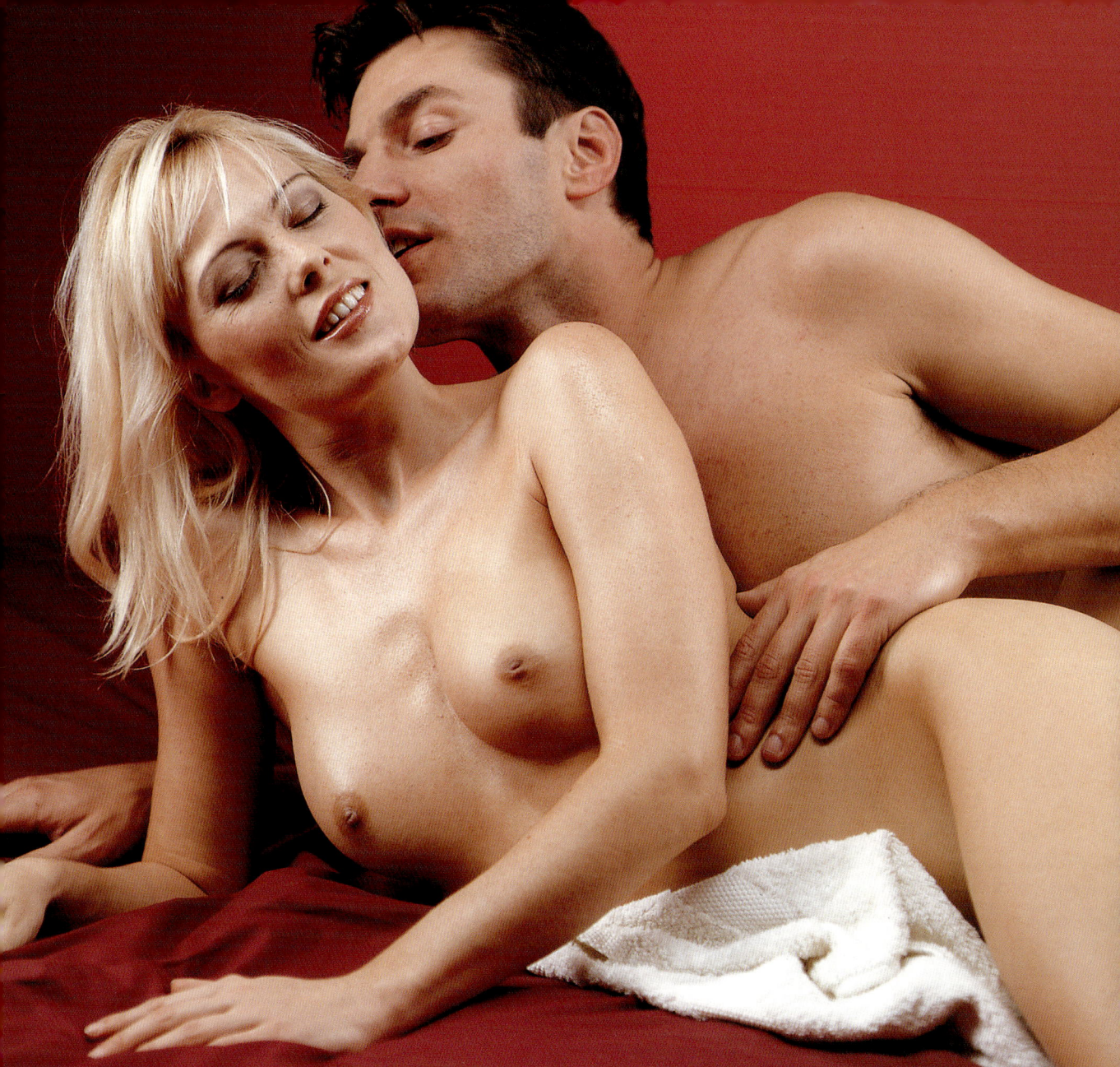

backs and wrists. Apply a little more of the oil to your palm, rub your hands together, then spread your hands and bring them down gently, lightly touching the skin, and begin to apply it using long slow strokes. Look to maintain continuous contact wherever possible.

Health enquiry

It is possible that your proposed massage partner may have health issues they have not yet revealed to you, for whatever reason. It is vital, however, that you get a clear answer on whether or not your partner has high or low blood pressure, suffers allergic skin reactions (if so, don't use essential oils or trigger products), has – or is – suffering from a prolapsed disc, a serious back problem or a heart condition (in which case, limit the sequences you use to those that avoid strain). If in doubt, use a non-allergenic talc or plain (not nut-based) carrier oils and avoid massage techniques that require strong manipulation (such as those in the chapter *Beyond Skin Deep*). If your partner is pregnant, use only light, sensitive strokes around her abdomen.

Getting into the mood

The key to giving a good sensual, erotic massage is sensitivity. Being attuned and responsive to your partner's feelings and needs – sexual or otherwise – will enhance the massage tenfold and increase the loving intimacy between you.

Synchronize your breathing

The massage giver may initiate a technique and direct a sequence, but the real goal is empathetic sensitivity. Many strokes have a rhythmic and repetitious flow to them. The art of the true masseur is to link those strokes to the recipient's breathing. If you can successfully synchronize your breathing with your partner's then, with sensitivity, match your strokes and physical movements to the rhythm of your mutual breath, a magic alchemy ensues, an almost mystical bonding of soul and spirit, when two become one.

Yoga bodywork

In the early stages, as you build your confidence and repertoire, what you do might seem rather artificial. Don't worry. With practice and the use of synchronized breath, balanced posture and one-pointed concentration on the needs of your partner, you are carrying out a form of yoga bodywork. This will have lasting health benefits for you and your fortunate partner. As with all acts of selfless giving, the rewards come back to the giver. Even if your partner is more egocentric than you, your generosity and kindness will help your personal growth, even if your partner seems to be the main beneficiary.

Therapy

Your partner may naturally wish to talk to release the mental and emotional burden of daily cares. This is usually only a temporary or short-lived habit that will quieten eventually. Sometimes the source of this is nervousness caused by insecurities or feelings of inadequacy.

Communication

Communication is King (and Queen!) when it comes to massage. Throughout a session you might elicit a bewildering range of reactions. Some exclamations might suggest your partner is in pain or discomfort when he or she is not (unless it is a pleasurable pain) while others may be genuine cries of distress. You need to know which is which. Establish a "safe word" in advance that means "stop what you are doing now." Doing this provides a secure backstop that gives partners the confidence to experiment and express themselves without restraint.

Fantasy and role play

It is not uncommon to have an erotic fantasy borrowed from a book or movie screen. As you become confident in your erotic exploration you might care to re-create a scenario, in word or action, which tickles your imagination. Learning to explore and express those desires is all part of building confidence and trust in each other. In case you're concerned, you're unlikely to be the only deviant on the planet!

Dress code

Just because you are going to give or enjoy an erotic massage, don't assume that it has to be nude. Attractive, comfortable, sexy clothes or underwear that make you feel good are really erotic and add extra flavor to role-play games.

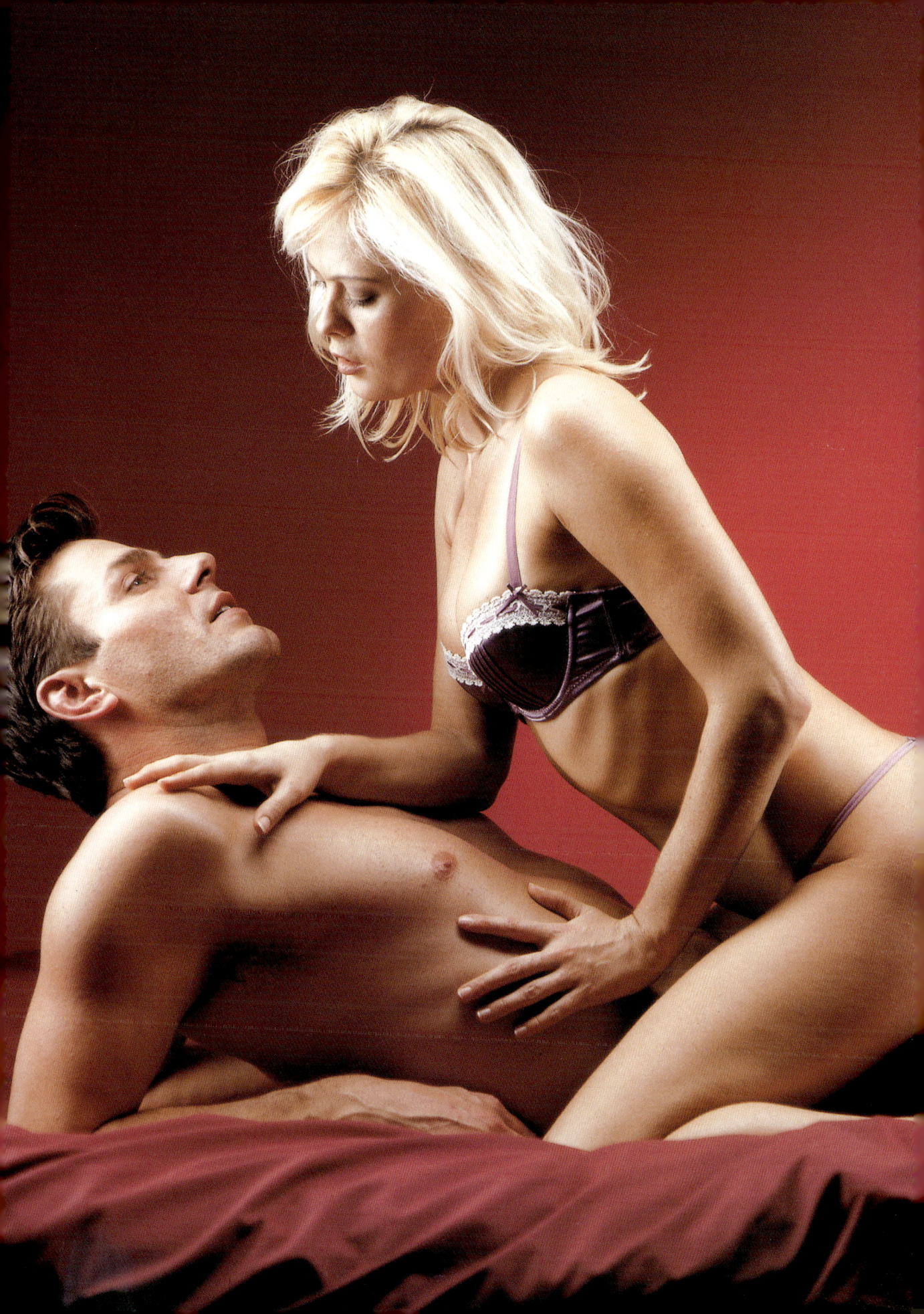

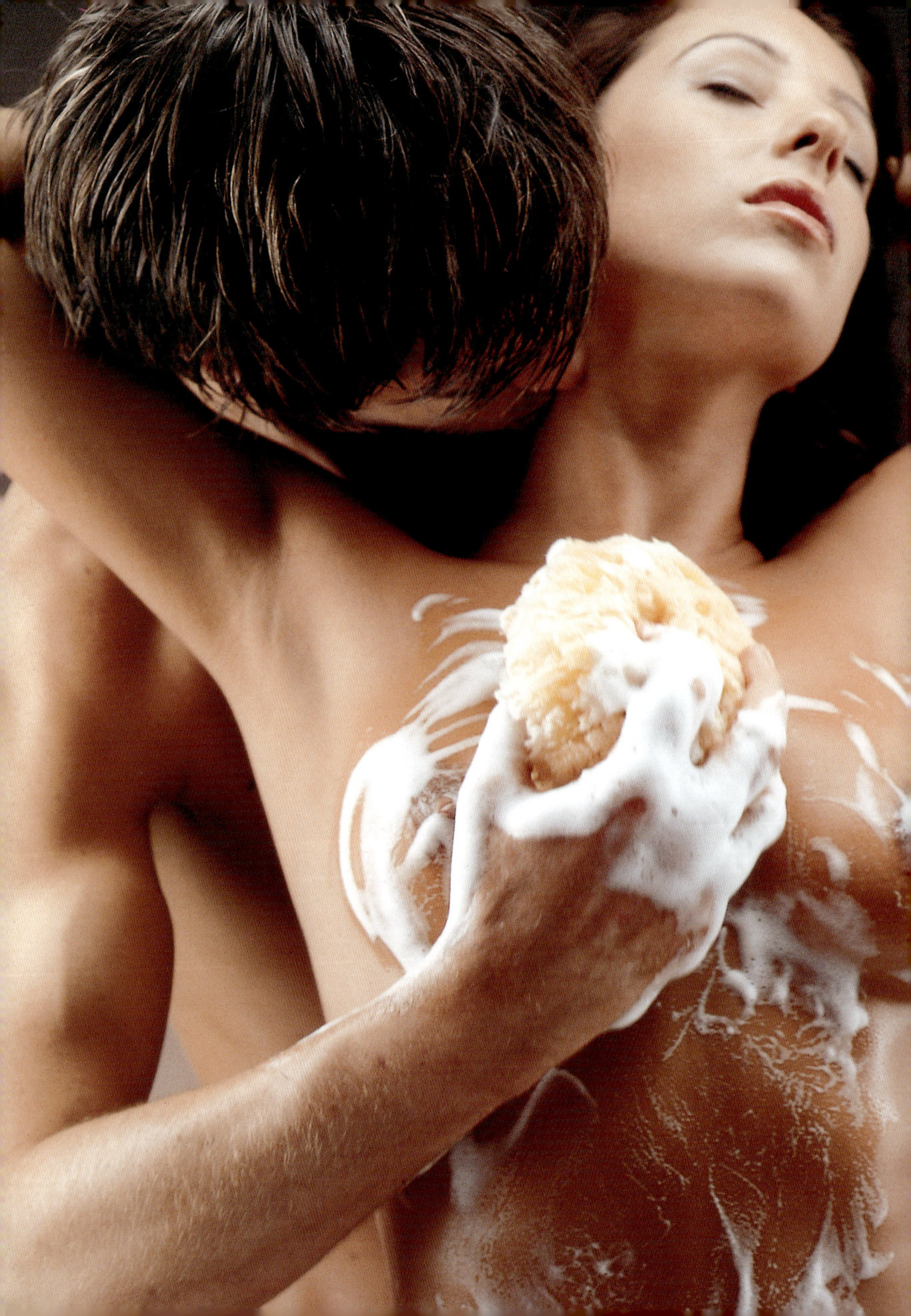

Get fresh

Sexy showers prepare the body for massage, while pampering cleansing routines soften the skin, ready for applying sensuous oils.

Sensual cleansing

There is nothing more sexy than vibrant skin that has shine and luster. With regular massage and care the skin is less likely to age and will have a greater elasticity. Healthy skin even makes the whole body appear to be more fluid in its movements.

Sexy showers

A refreshing and cleansing shower is a great way to prepare for an erotic massage. Why a shower rather than a bath? Well, a bath is less a perfunctory or obligatory chore than a luxurious sybaritic delight to be savored while you are in a dreamy alpha state. A shower, psychologically, suggests a washing away of all detritus and negativity. It demarcates between your state of being or way of working before your shower and the state you get into for and during your erotic massage, and so reduces the mental and emotional baggage you bring into the massage. Showering also prepares you for a new "rule set" – it signifies that a new way of being can now occur, that certain conventions of dress and restrained behavior need not necessarily apply for a while.

If you can be with your massage partner, a shared shower is an excellent way to set expectations, sometimes play out fantasies and, conversely, get down and dirty! With that in mind, below are three recipes that will help to cleanse and refresh the body.

Rub-a-dub scrub

For a natural and effective exfoliator, mix together sea salt and almond oil to form a rich paste. Then, using a natural loofah, a shower glove or your bare hands, scoop up handfuls of the rich scrub and rub over dry areas of the body, such as the upper arms, elbows, thighs, buttocks and lower legs. This removes any dead skin cells while softening and refreshing the skin and, by bringing the blood vessels to the surface, it leaves the skin feeling more sensitive and invigorated.

Coconut milk skin tonic

It feels extravagant and naughty to use milk like an elixir for eternal youth. If your skin is not in the best condition you'll go nuts for this tonic – it literally leaves your skin glowing like silk. Simply mix together two to three cups of organic coconut milk, warm in a saucepan and decant into a flask, ready for use. Rub over the skin while you're in the shower. Leave the tonic on for a few minutes, then shower off.

Papaya body polish

For extra polish, apply very ripe mashed papaya over the body, especially around the eyes, face and neck to keep wrinkles at bay. Allow the mashed papaya to dry, then shower off.

Psychic shower

If it is not possible to take a physical shower before your massage, you might try a psychic one. Imagine you are standing under a crystal-clear waterfall. As it flows over head and body, all those negative particles, worries and concerns are being washed away. Alternatively, "cleanse" your body by smoothing your hands over its surface with firm pressure, as if wiping off raindrops or a slick of grease, making sure you cover every inch. "Flick" the surplus off your hands to cleanse yourself of negative energy.

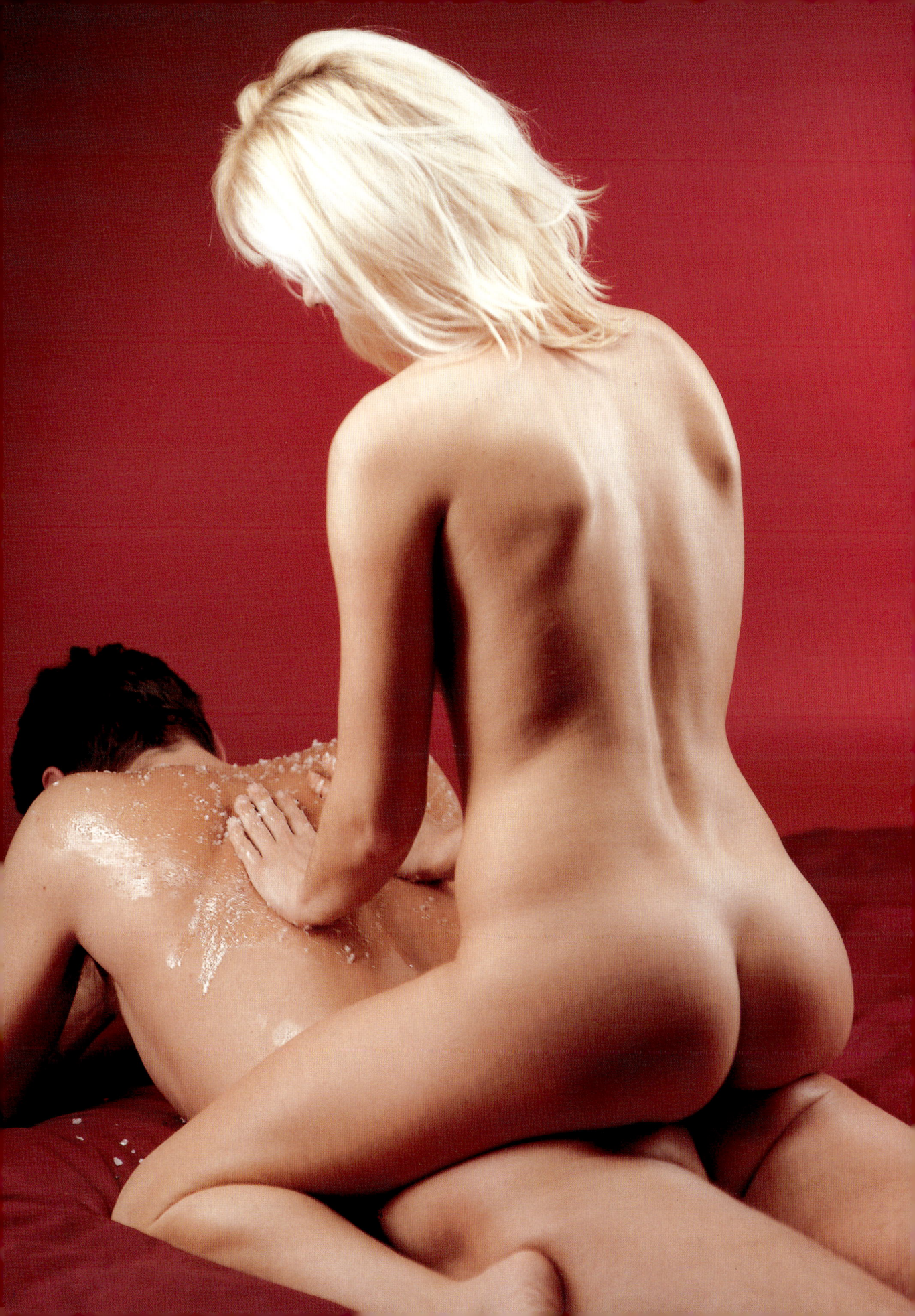

Drying the skin

Drying is frequently done in a rush or absent-mindedly after a bath or shower, and its potential for pleasure and arousal is all too often neglected. But there is no reason why drying each other's skin shouldn't be a thoroughly sensual experience. Drying is an integral part of the loving ritual of bathing, and this is an ideal opportunity to explore and get to know one another's body more intimately.

Blow drying

After your shower you're going to want to dry your bodies. Be sure to have large fluffy towels waiting, but you might also consider some drying fun with hair dryers. These handy tools, deftly wielded, can deliver a full spectrum of sensations, from the lightest of warm breezes to sensitive areas to hot and cold intensity on any surface for startling effect. When used on the head it is reminiscent of the pampering care lavished on you by your hairdresser – a time when your needs are at the center of attention.

Bit of rough

Not everyone is looking for soft pampering. Sometimes the opposite is true. Try drying the skin with old, rough towels that stimulate the skin surface. On hot days you could enjoy the frisson of chilled towels pre-cooled in the refrigerator in plastic bags.

You do me, I'll do you

We all have our own style of drying ourselves – some ways are more methodical or efficient than others. If you exchange drying duties with your partner you can learn about his or her approach to life. This is another way of getting to know a new partner – or rediscovering a familiar one.

Baby powder

When you were a baby, the chances are that after bathing your body would receive a liberal dusting of talcum powder. It is one of those evocative babyhood memories that reminds us of a time when we were cherished and loved and the object of everyone's adoration. Baby powder is also an alternative to oiling the body as a means of reducing friction prior to a massage stroke or routine. If you plan to wear expensive or delicate clothing (however skimpy) you may have a concern that essential oils might stain and damage your garments. If you take pride in your home or have an especial care for the place you plan to carry out your fun and games, then similar considerations might apply.

Not everyone has clear, unblemished and tolerant skin. Some of you may be sensitive to the active ingredients in even the safest of plant-based oils. Talc has the advantage of coming in non-allergenic form or perfumed with a favorite or complementary scent. Applied with a cotton ball or pad applicator the fun and games of drying and baby powder are a great way to break down inhibitions and create a relaxed atmosphere between a couple. Also, reddened, cut or bruised flesh is de-emphasized as the foundation-like application of talc creates a smooth, soft skin surface.

drying the skin should be a thoroughly sensual experience

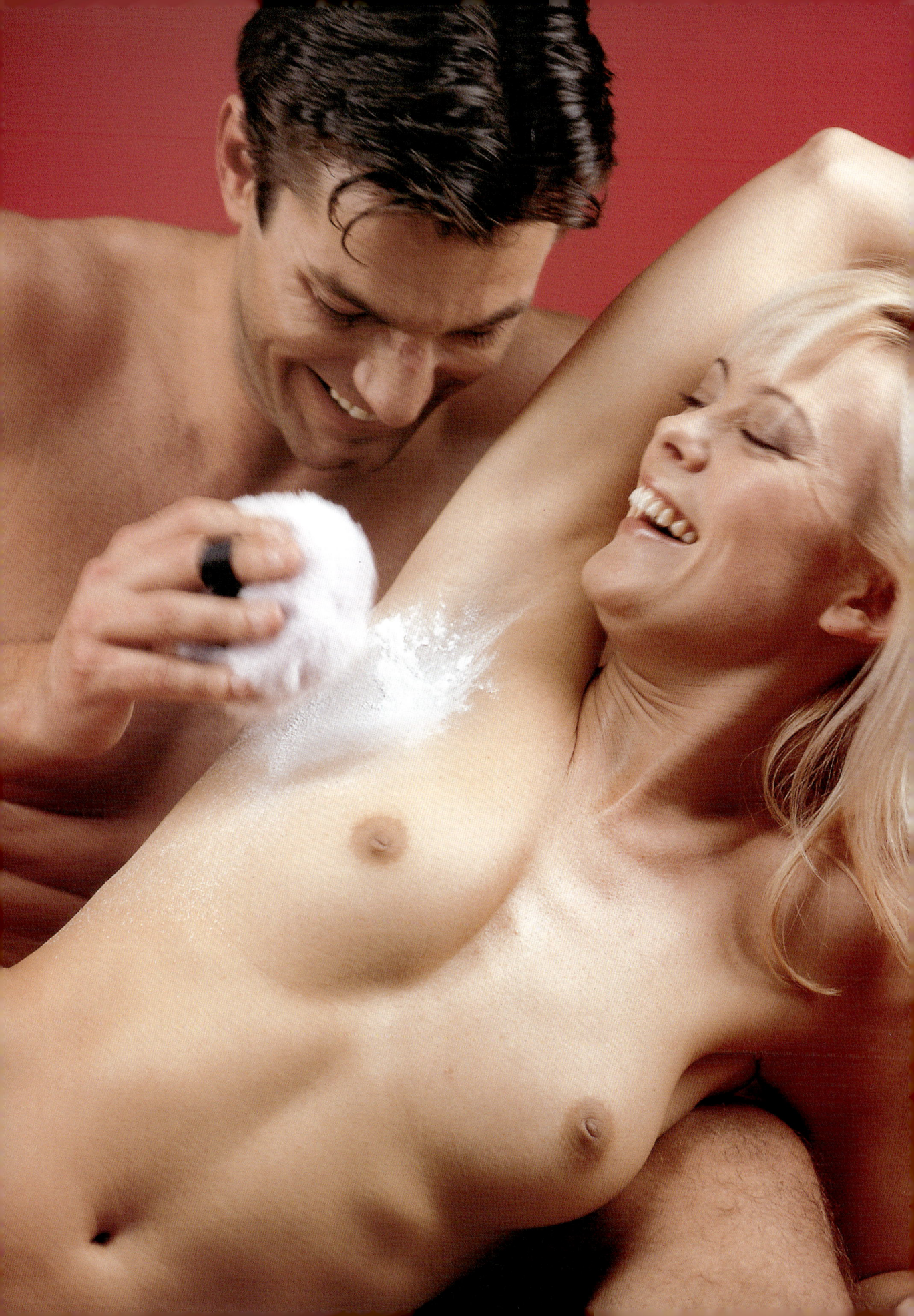

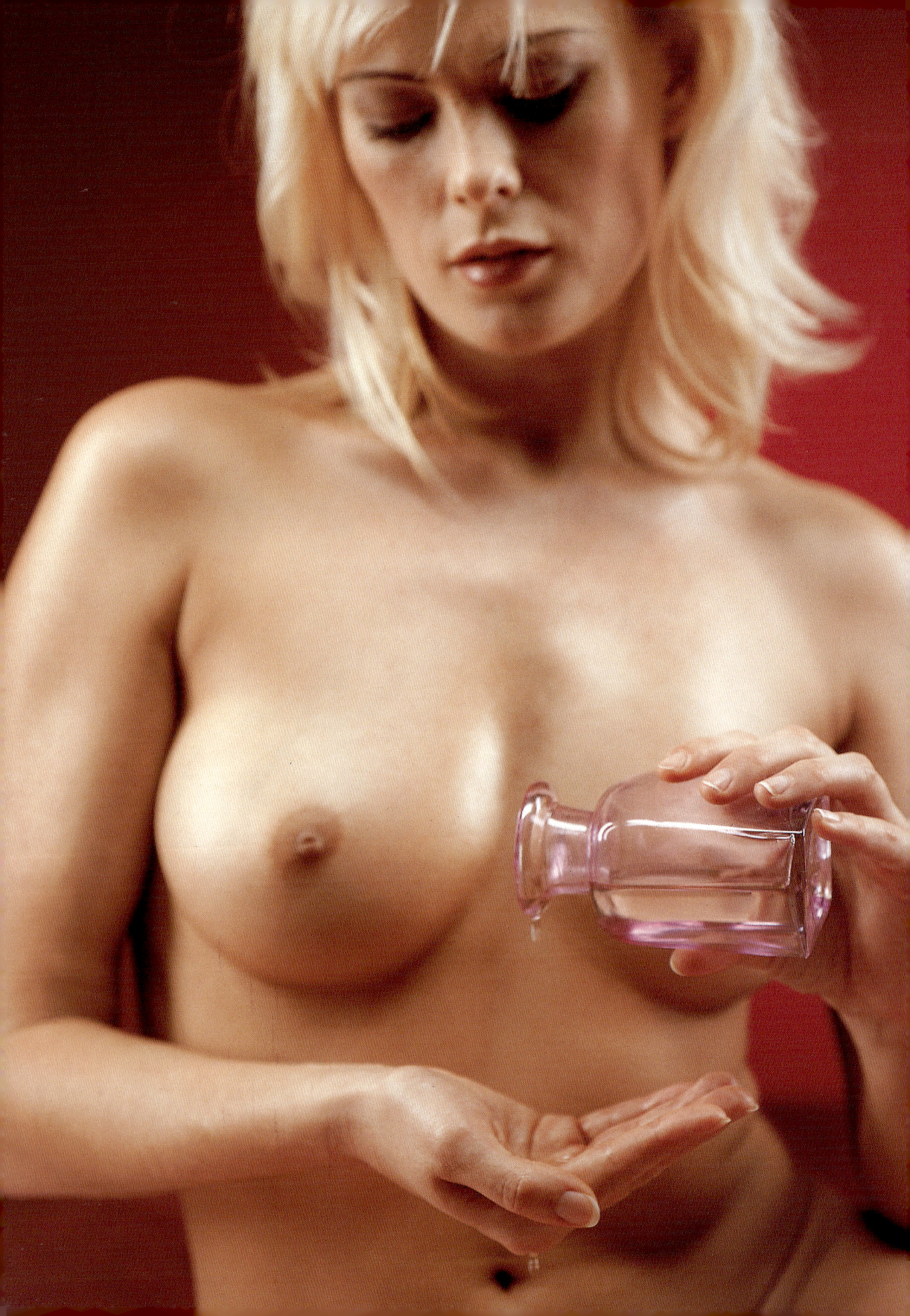

Oils and lotions

Massage requires a suitable form of lubrication to avoid causing friction or chafing the skin with the movement of the hands. The traditional media for massage are oils or lotions.

Oils and aromatherapy

Clearly the viscous, petroleum-based motor oils and low-grade heavy cooking oils are not appropriate for massage use! Light oils such as sweet almond or safflower are the base or carrier oils of choice. A base or carrier oil has little or no smell, and can be used alone or blended with an essential oil to give it its smell and therapeutic properties. An essential oil is a plant extract with active medicinal properties. There is a broad range of essential oils available, each with its own properties that you can utilize. There are plenty of books that describe their properties and individual cautions. You can select one to match a physical condition you wish to treat, or simply choose a scent that appeals to you. Alternatively, simply choose your favorite smell.

A standard measuring teaspoon holds exactly 100 drops of oil. Most essential oils are used in a safe three percent solution. This means three drops of essential oil should be added to a one teaspoon of carrier oil. Obviously, one spoonful is not enough for an average adult massage so we'd recommend the following proportions: for a small adult, add six drops of essential oil to two teaspoons carrier oil; for a medium-sized adult, add seven to eight drops per three tablespoons; for a large adult, add nine to ten drops per four teaspoons. If you run out of blended treatment oil, supplement it with as much plain carrier oil as required. Using this essential oil/carrier oil ratio, you can create your own mixes, although it is advisable to give your partner the chance to smell the available options to be sure he or she likes the scents available.

There are a few simple guidelines that amateur aromatherapists should follow. Ensure you have plenty of oil mix handy. Although you're only looking to impart a thin, even layer of lubrication to aid your gliding massage strokes, sometimes dry and under-nourished skin can absorb quite a quantity of oil and a hairy man needs greater lubrication to ensure comfort. Take care not to work your oiled hands too close to the body's sensitive orifices (eyes, nostrils, anus or vulva) as the active ingredients may cause irritation.

Lotion in motion

Lotions are an excellent choice for massage since they are largely non-sticky, light and easily absorbed into the skin. Plus, the chances are that your or your partner's favorite scent has a lotion in its range. Designed for larger areas of skin coverage, they are diluted to safe levels and suitable for general use.

Cautions

If you suffer from a nut allergy, make sure you use a nut-free carrier oil such as safflower oil. When choosing essential oils, read the cautions relating to each oil before purchase. Many can be dangerous for use during pregnancy, while others should be avoided by people suffering from conditions such as high blood pressure. If in doubt about a product, either ask the supplier or an aromatherapist or, in the absence of reliable advice, opt for an oil that you know to be safe.

Sensual scents

As an alternative to commercial oil mixes, create a custom mix based on your preferred scent and product type, including everything from perfume, eau de toilette and spritzers to body lotion, shower gel, soap and talc – this is where you can get creative. For instance, in hot weather a lightly chilled spritzer spray can be a deliciously tantalizing prelude to a massage and will leave a scent trail for the carrier oil, applied on top of it, to pick up. Or an eau de toilette might be sprayed lightly on to the body after oiling with a plain carrier oil.

You might consider asking your partner to bring a spray version of his or her favorite scent. Conventional wisdom suggests a woman is better advised to choose her own scent for herself rather than let her partner loose in a department store! Conversely, women sometimes have sure instincts for their mate although they should remember that a lot of men are conservative and predictable in their choices. If things go horribly wrong, have a fairly neutral or non-offensive standby on hand, and remember that it is always possible to quickly shower off and start again in the event of a disaster. Men, by reputation, seem to prefer and suit woody, spicy and earthy tones.

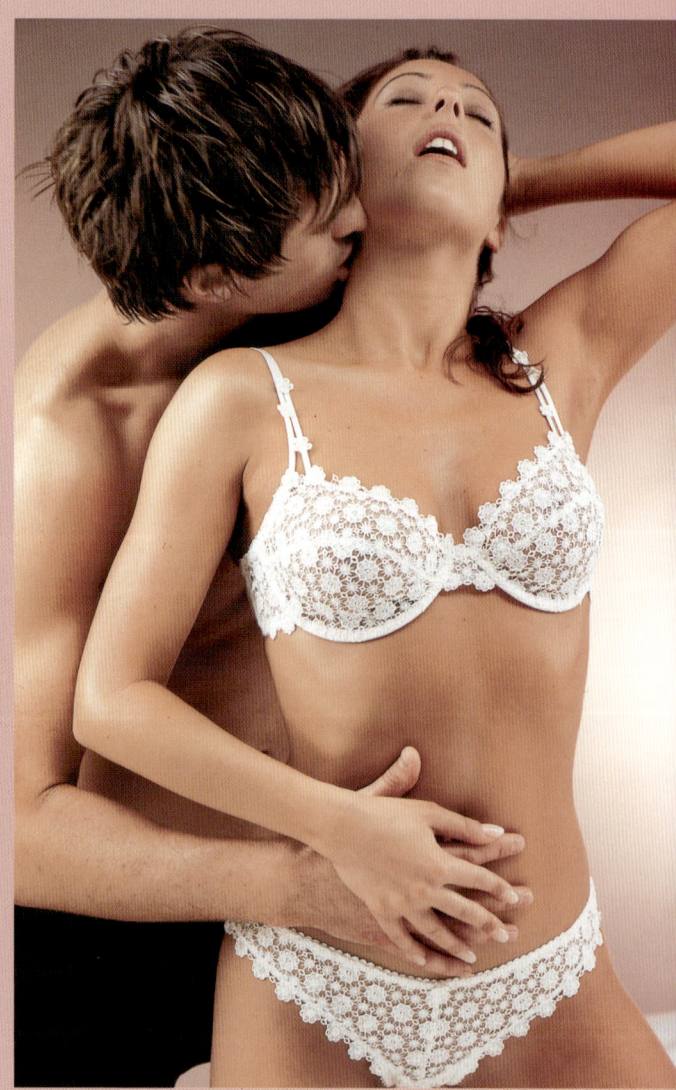

Hot tip
If you plan to indulge in kissing and licking, bear in mind that some mixes can taste bitter or unpleasant. Try the "taste test." Spray a little of your chosen scent on your forearm, then rub a drop of carrier oil on top. Kiss the skin for a foretaste of what your partner will taste and, hopefully, enjoy. All perfumes have ingredients that are bitter or musky and benefit from being diluted by a swig of champagne or other drink.

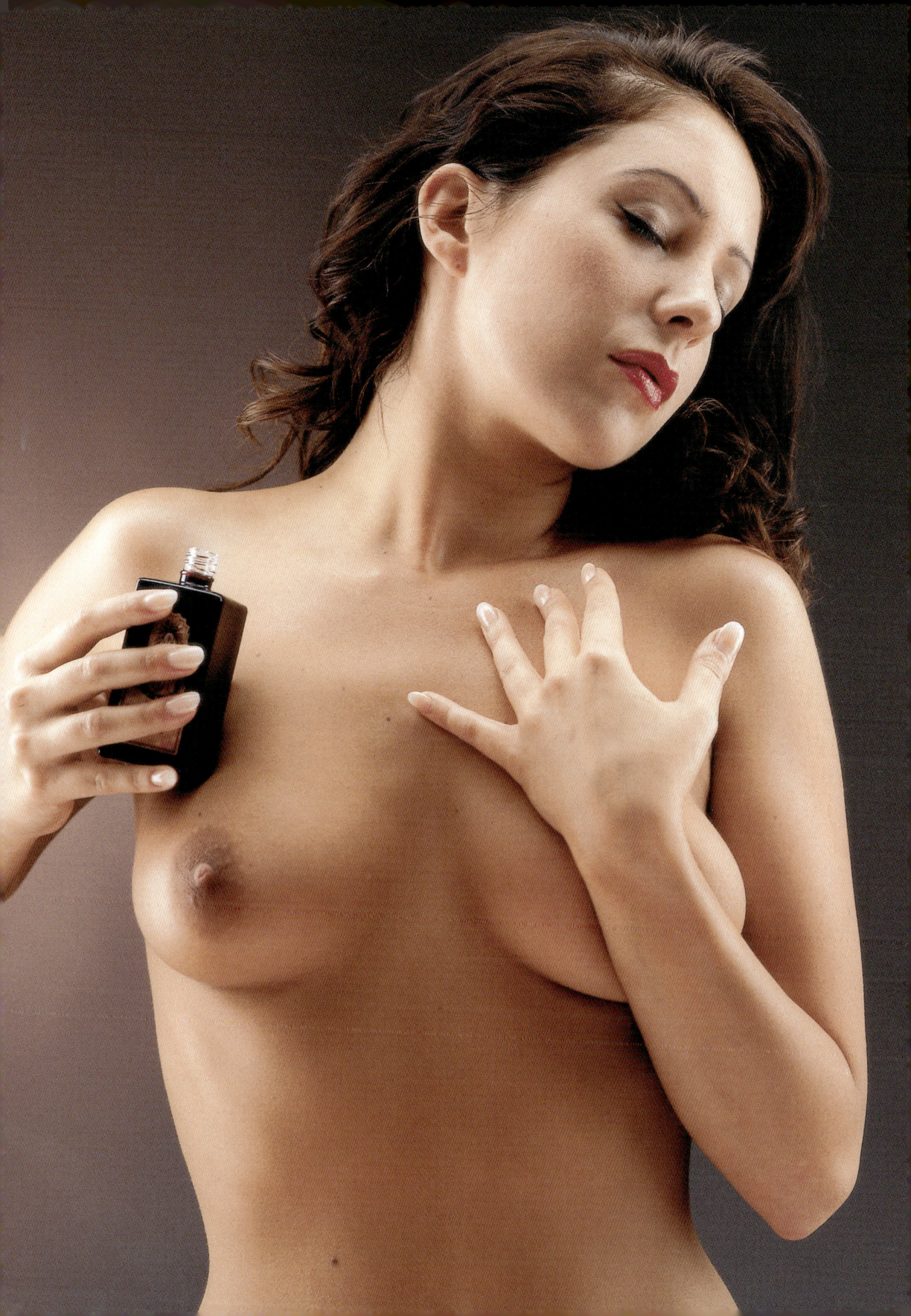

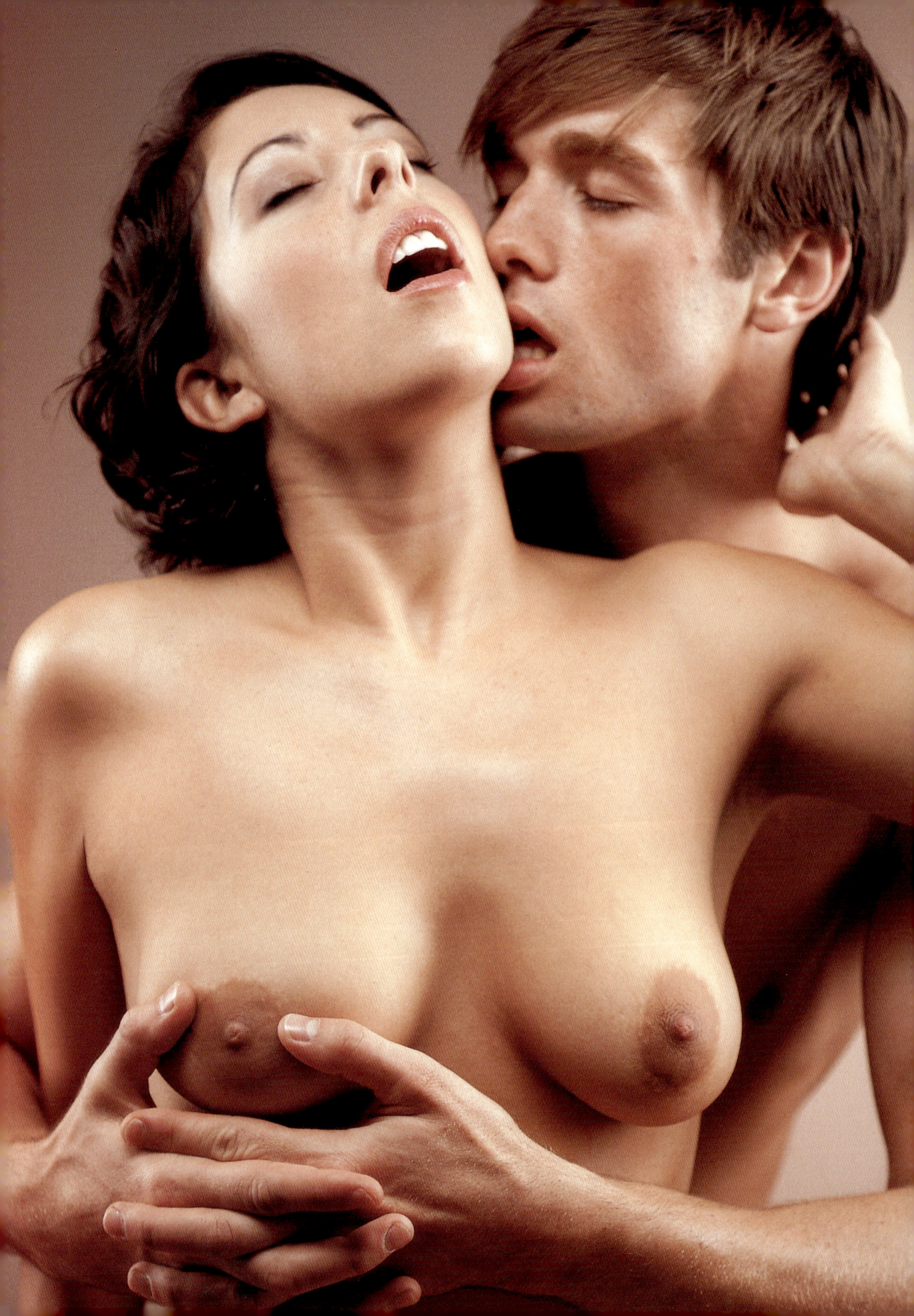

Pleasure zones

Explore and indulge the erotic palate with subtle tongue tricks and gentle feathering, circling and effleurage strokes.

Face, ears and scalp

The sequences in this chapter can form part of a complete massage (used in the order in which they appear) or any of them can be used as a prelude to another sequence from the book. Sitting either cross-legged or kneeling, place a cushion in your lap or on your thighs and invite your partner to lie on his back, with head resting on the cushion.

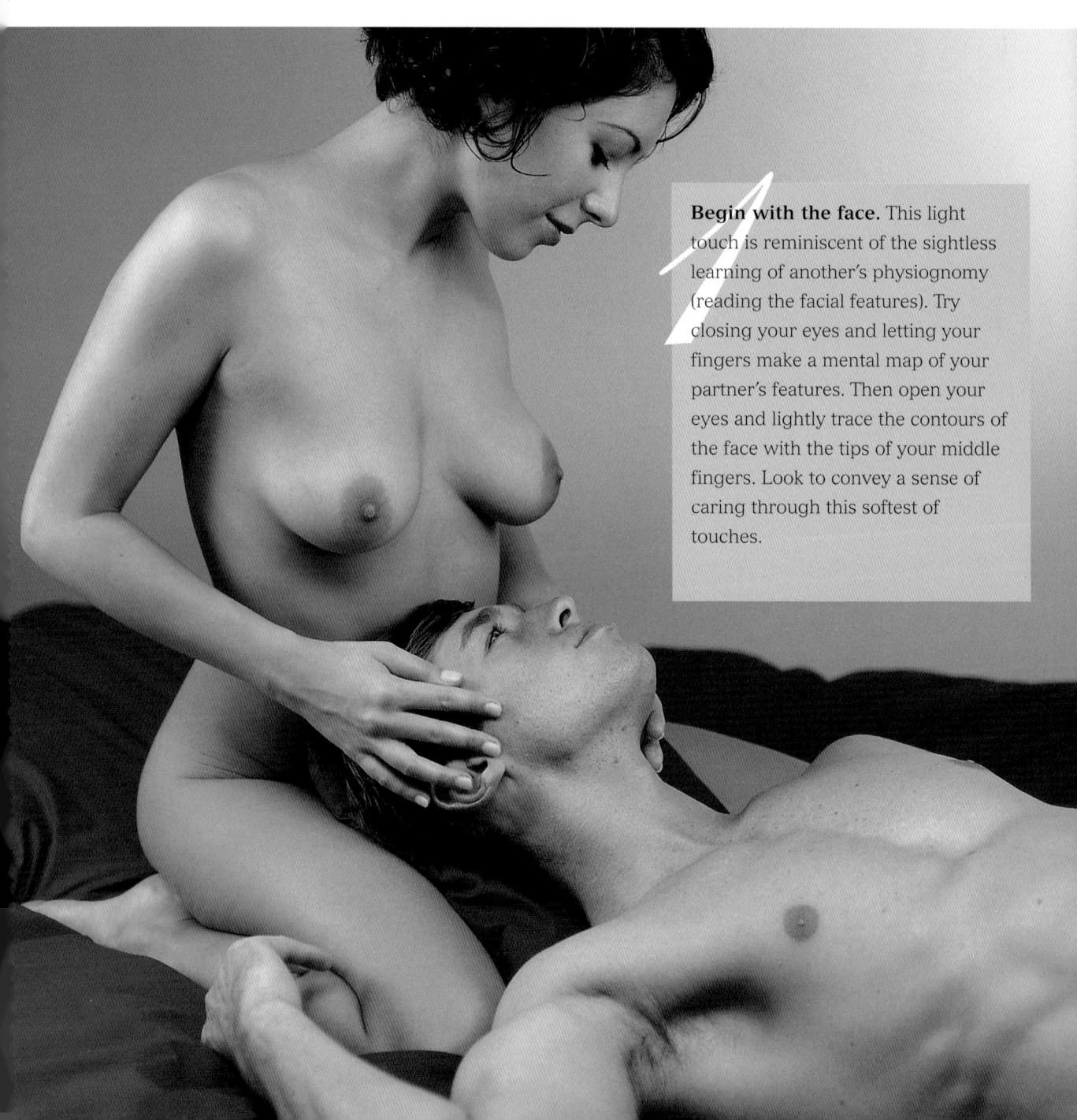

1 Begin with the face. This light touch is reminiscent of the sightless learning of another's physiognomy (reading the facial features). Try closing your eyes and letting your fingers make a mental map of your partner's features. Then open your eyes and lightly trace the contours of the face with the tips of your middle fingers. Look to convey a sense of caring through this softest of touches.

Move on to the ears. Like the feet, the ears contain many acupuncture points and meridians. They are both sensitive and sensual. Place each ear between a thumb and forefinger and squeeze along the edges by making small circular movements with gentle pressure. Gently pluck and pull the edges of the ears and finish off with a light pull downward on the ear lobes. For a truly sensual treat, trace the inner crevices of the ears with your tongue and breathe warmly into them.

Begin the scalp massage by stroking the hair. Then, with one or both hands, grasp a bunch of hair close to the scalp and either make gentle circular movements with your wrist or pull the hair toward you with care. Release your grasp and glide your fingers upward toward the crown in a gentle raking movement. Repeat using alternate hands. This technique gives a great sense of relief by "pulling away" the tightness in the scalp. Try scratching the scalp for a different reaction – perhaps a shiver of delight down the backbone!

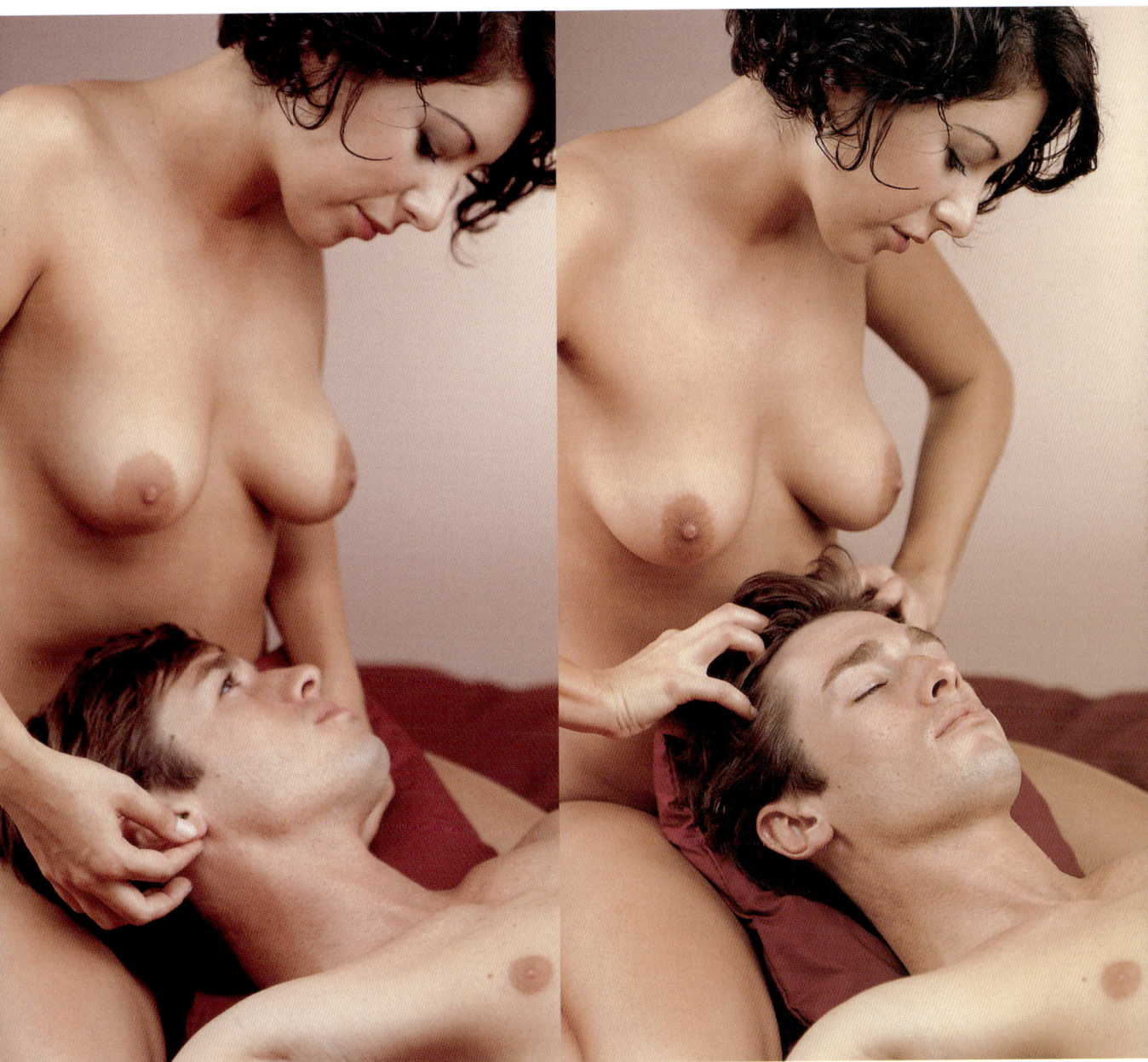

Face, ears and scalp

Temples, lips and neck

Remain in the seated position with your partner's head resting on your lap for this part of the sequence. The temple massage helps to clear the mind and focus on the moment, while the ideas for touching the lips and neck are highly arousing.

1 To massage the temples, cradle your partner's head in your hands and circle the temples lightly with the middle fingers. Cup the ears with your palms for a minute to help your partner forget about the cares of the outside world and internalize the consciousness – to listen to the beat of his heart and the musical sound of the blood moving. This technique provides ideal therapy for those with over-busy minds.

2 Trace in and around the lips with the fingertips or the nipples. There are so many nerve endings in the lips that even the subtlest of touches can be felt. In fact, the lighter the touch on any part of the body, the more sensitized the whole body becomes. Set "soft and gentle" as the tone for your massage at the start, making it easier to avoid becoming heavy-handed later on in the sequence.

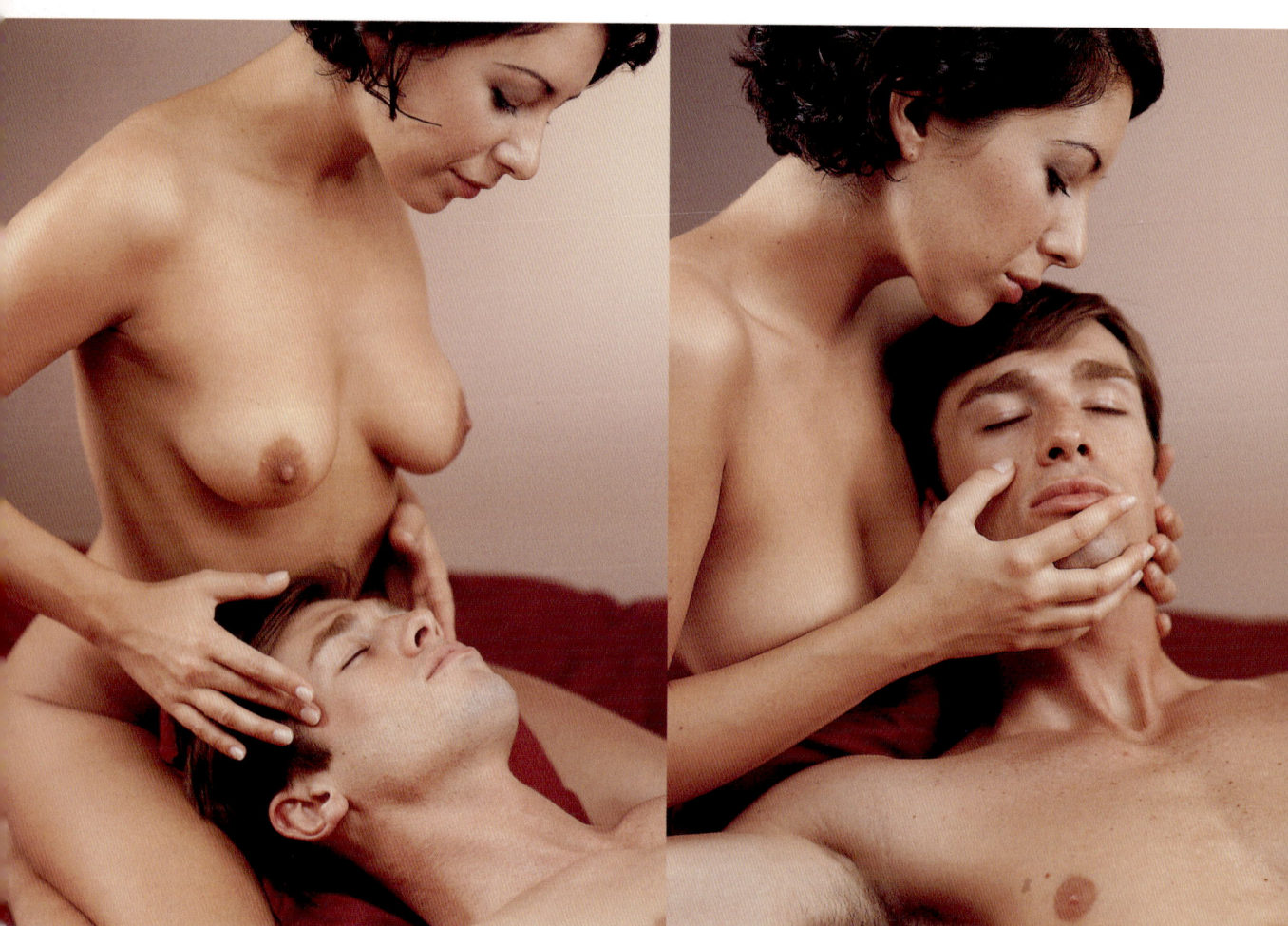

28   Pleasure zones

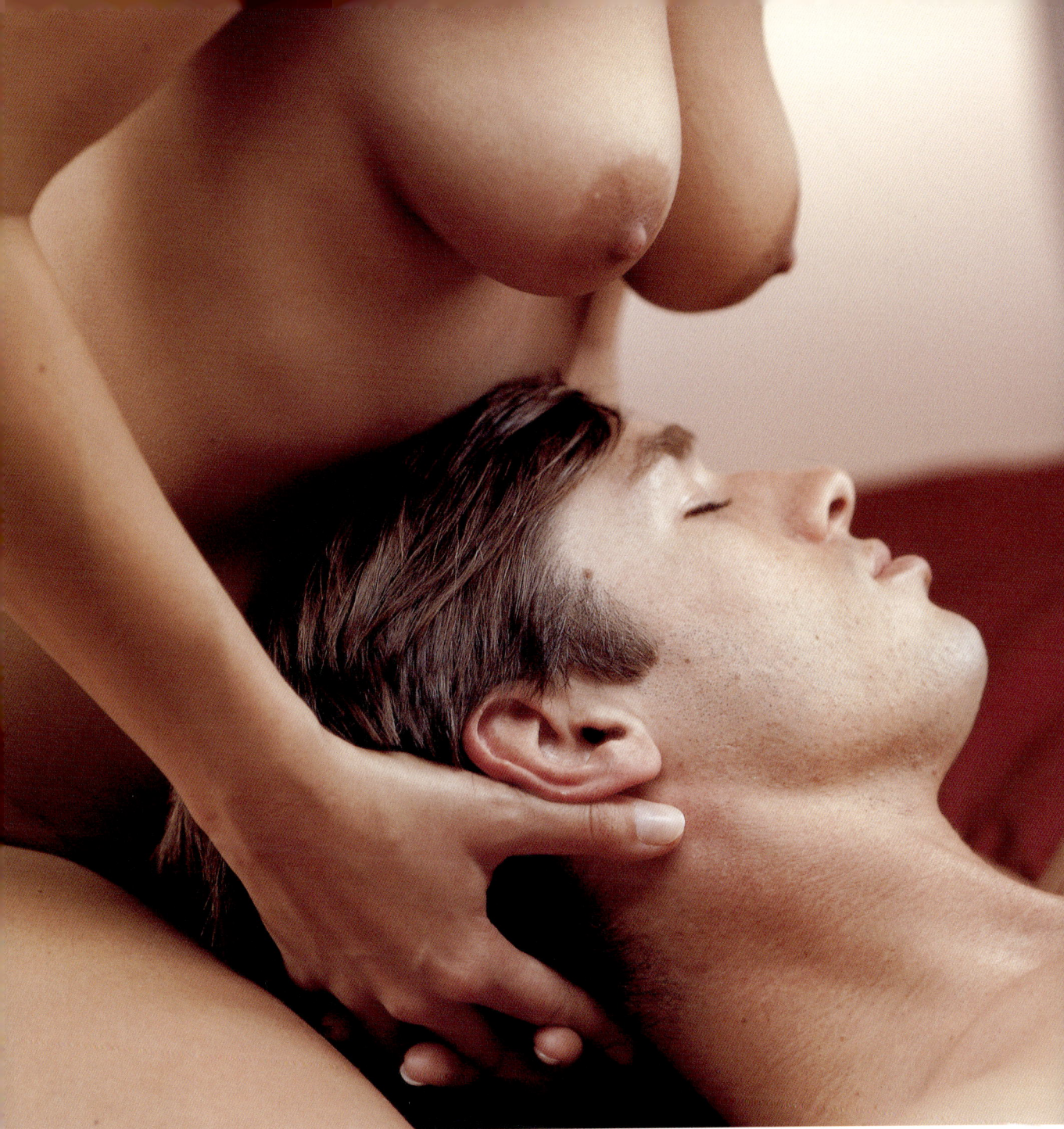

A slight pull on the neck can ease a lot of tension. Slip your hands under the back of the neck and interlace your fingers. Slowly and gently ease the neck toward you, pulling gently and using the power of the clasped hands to exert a delicate but considered pressure against the base of the skull. Release slowly and repeat the movement six times.

Hot tip
Rake the fingers up the back of the neck and through the scalp, working along all your partner's sensitive areas, especially behind the ears, and stroking the hair at the base of the skull.

The chest

Ask your partner to stand up or kneel on the floor, then position yourself close behind her for this part of the massage. The nipples and breasts are highly erogenous zones for most women and for many men, too, although some men might not immediately appreciate the sensitivity of these areas. The following techniques can be used on both men and women.

Place the thumbs on either side of one nipple and, as if following the spokes of a wheel, gently and slowly glide your thumbs to the outer edges of a woman's breast, or toward the edges of the chest for approximately three inches on a man. Work your thumbs around the circle of each nipple.

Apply a light stroke over the breasts or chest with the fingers slightly splayed, allowing an erect nipple to get "caught" momentarily between the fingers, just before the hands are lifted off and another light stroke comes in from a different angle and on another path across the breast.

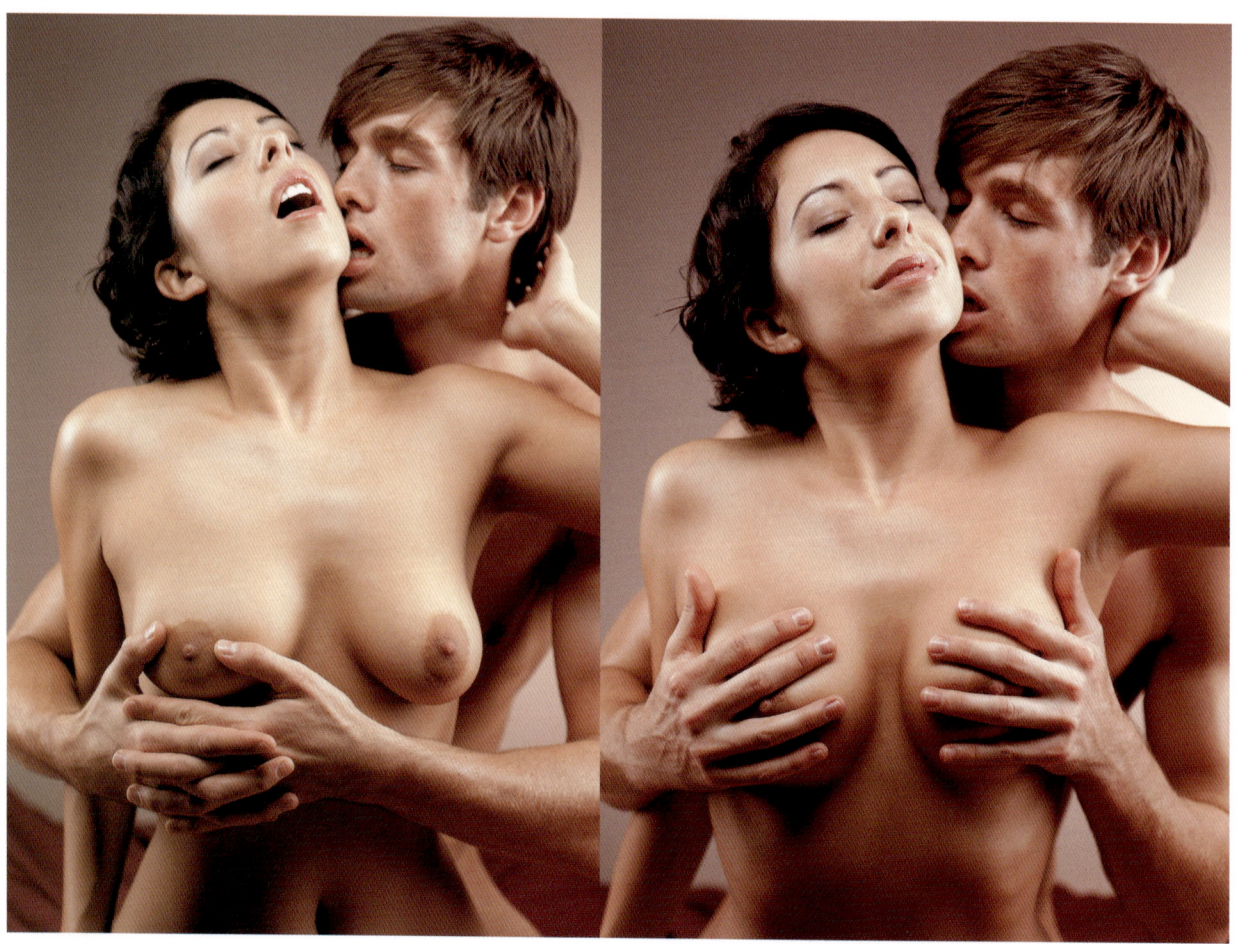

3 Lightly cup under the breasts and move in three clockwise or anti-clockwise circles, then stroke on and around the nipples with the middle fingers as a finishing touch. At any time, here and with other strokes and techniques, allow arms and hands to glide past "accidentally" or nonchalantly, merely grazing the breasts or nipples. This will have the subtle effect of linking highly sensitive erogenous zones to the rest of the body.

Hot tip
Warm your mouth with a hot drink before giving a quickie tongue massage to the nipples. Purse your lips as though blowing through a straw then slowly blow through the lips over sensitive areas.

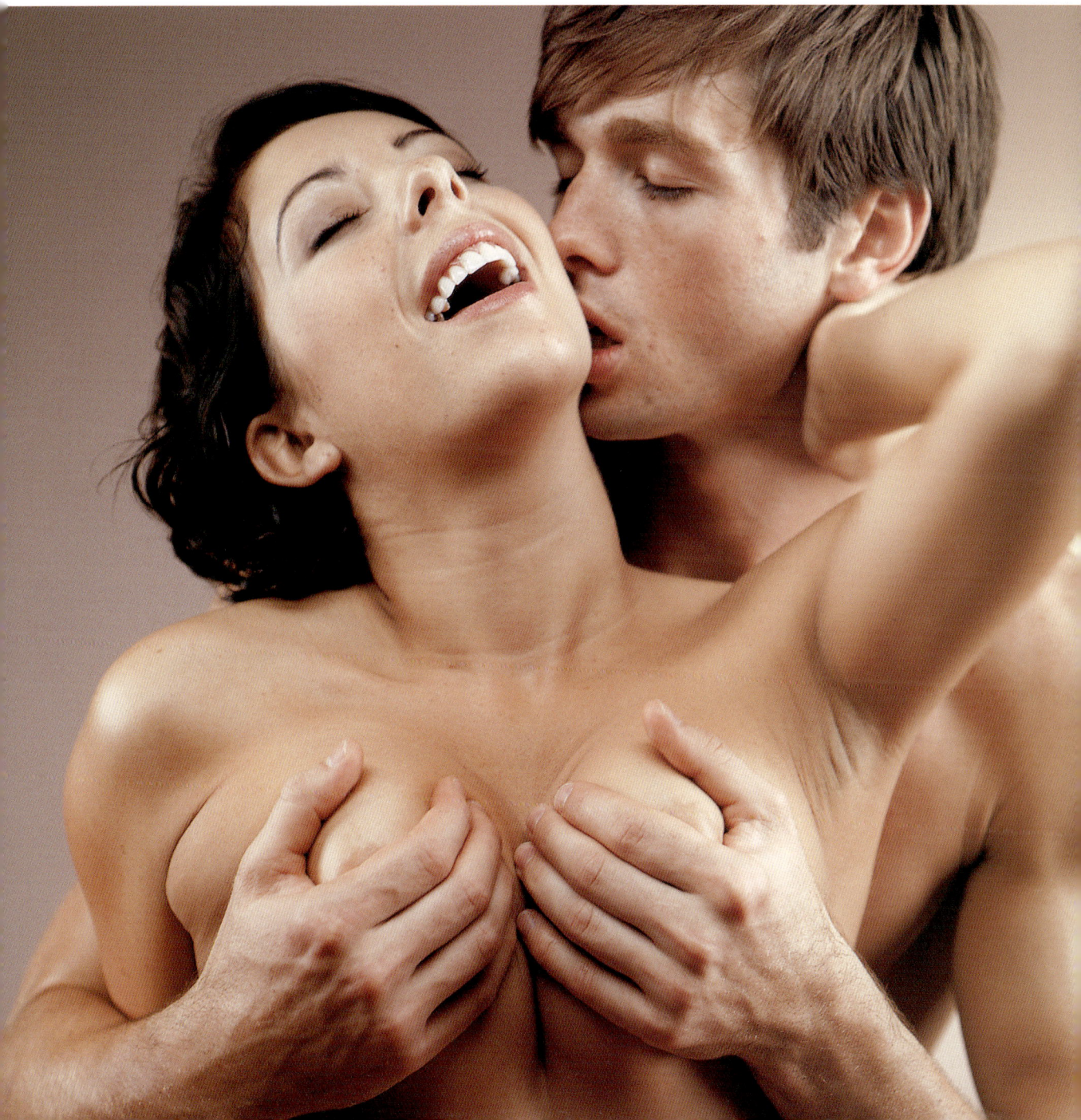

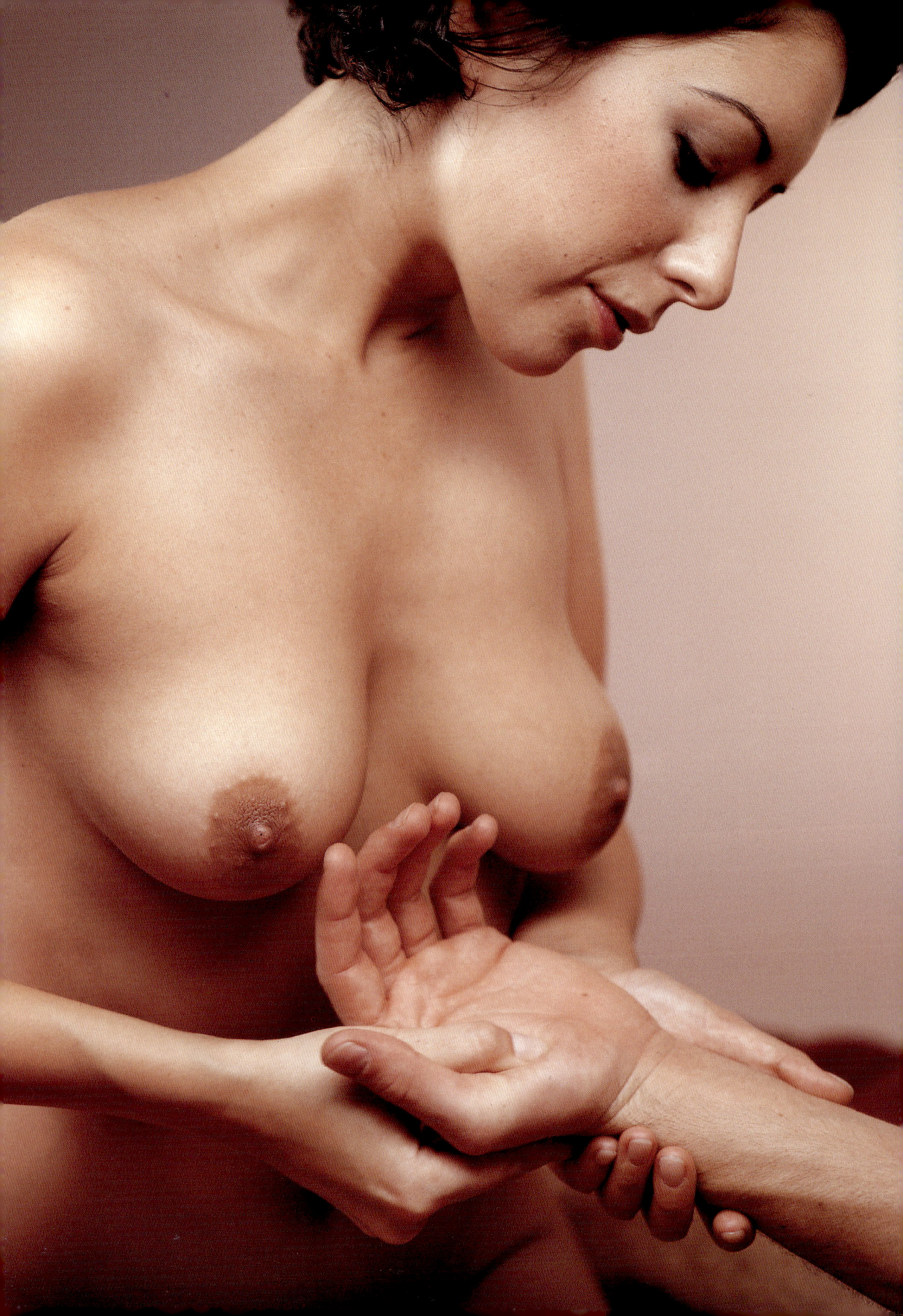

Palms and wrists

Sit beside your partner's hip or waist on either side of the body to perform this part of the massage. A great deal of tension – physical, emotional and mental – can be trapped in the hands, but they are often overlooked in massage. The following techniques can help to release this tension. As a prelude to the massage, softly trace the creases (head, heart and life lines) with your middle (heart) finger. Repeat this sequence on both hands.

1 Hold your partner's hand with both hands and rub the thumb of your working hand lightly over the palm and wrist in a small, circular motion, teasing and relaxing the fleshy bumps, such as the Mound of Venus (situated at the base of the thumb). As your thumbs press deeper into the flesh of the palm, note signs of stress release from your partner, particularly sighing, that indicate the efficacy of your treatment.

2 Feel your partner's pulse at the wrist. It can be readily located, but it requires a patient and attentive partner to feel it. Be aware that it is, literally, your partner's pulsing lifeblood. Count the pulse while gazing into your beloved's eyes. Place three fingers side-by-side just above the wrist joint, on the upper half of the wrist. This is the site of the diagnostic point called the Three Heater meridian – one of the master points for the subtle life energy that flows throughout our being. This point can reveal imbalance in the overall system and your careful and kind attention may help catalyze a change for the better. It is further rumored that an ancient Korean lovemaking tip is to gently tap this point in time with the pulse to bring your partner to orgasm.

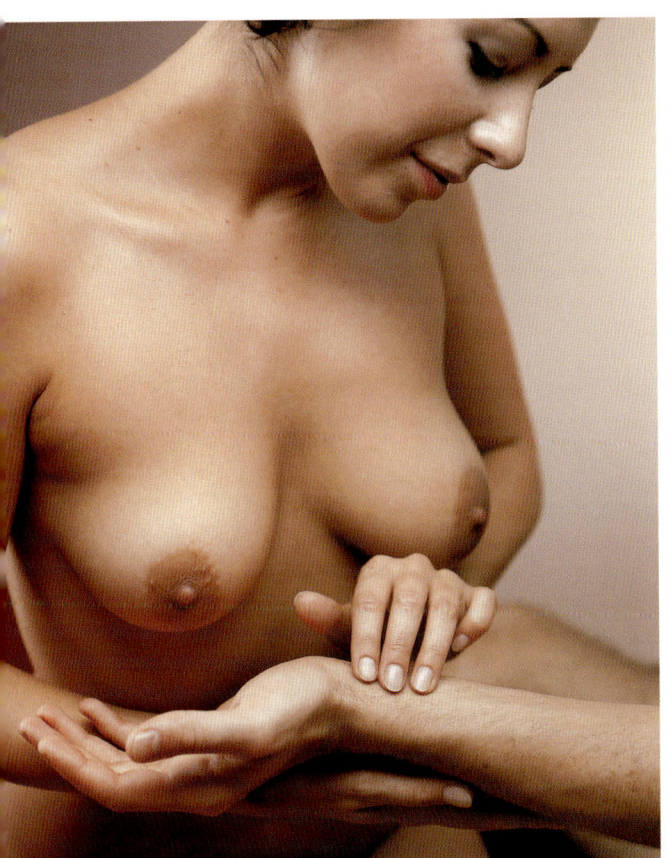

Hot tip
Synchronize your heartbeat and breath with your partner's by placing one palm on his heart (on the left side of his chest). Feel for the heartbeat and hold for long enough for your hearts to synchronize and create a loving empathy. Either gaze gently and lovingly into your partner's eyes, or close your eyes and "feel" with your fingers. After a few minutes stroke your hands down your partner's outstretched arm and finish by cradling his hand in both of yours, allowing your breath to fully synchronize with his.

The stomach

For this part of the sequence, ask your partner to lie down on her back and position yourself by the left side of the body. (If you are left-handed, you may prefer to be positioned on the right side, and use your left hand to perform the sequence.)

1 Place the back of your right hand flat against the center of the navel, bending your wrist so that your fingers point toward you, and pushing your elbow away from your body so that your forearm is upright. Now rotate your hand clockwise so that your fingers point toward the feet.

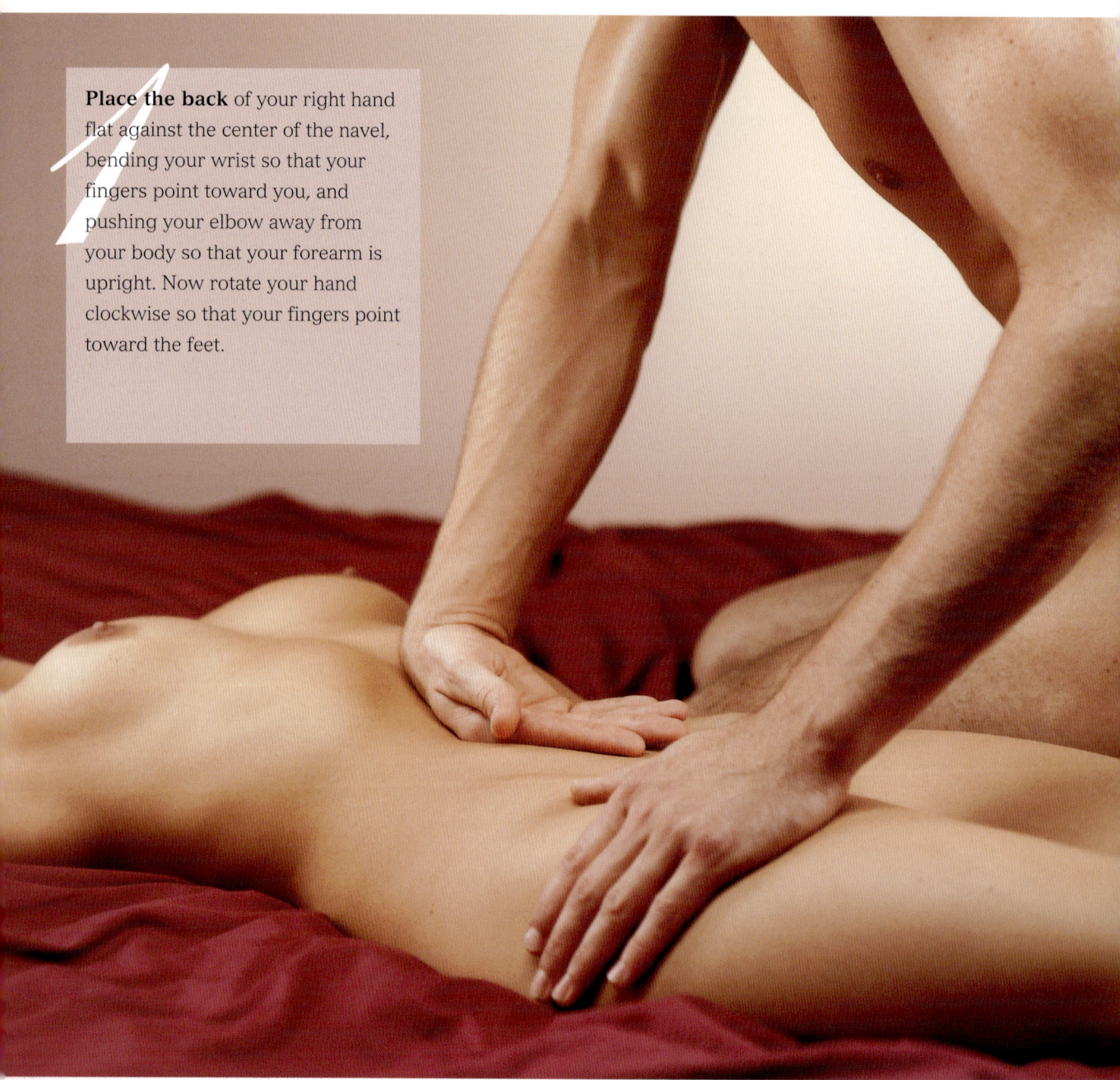

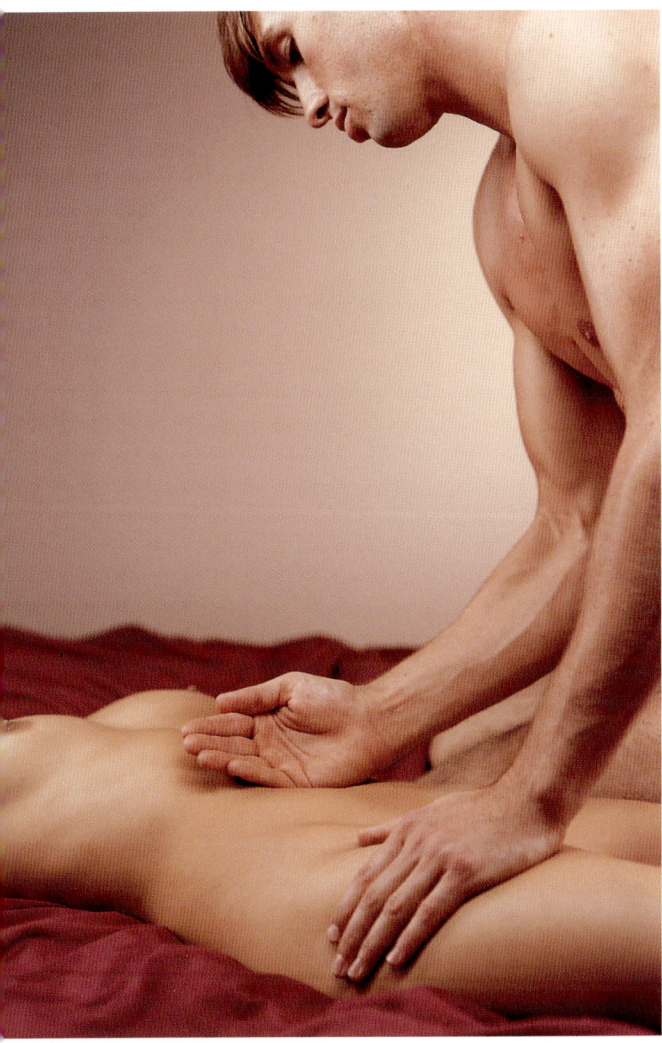 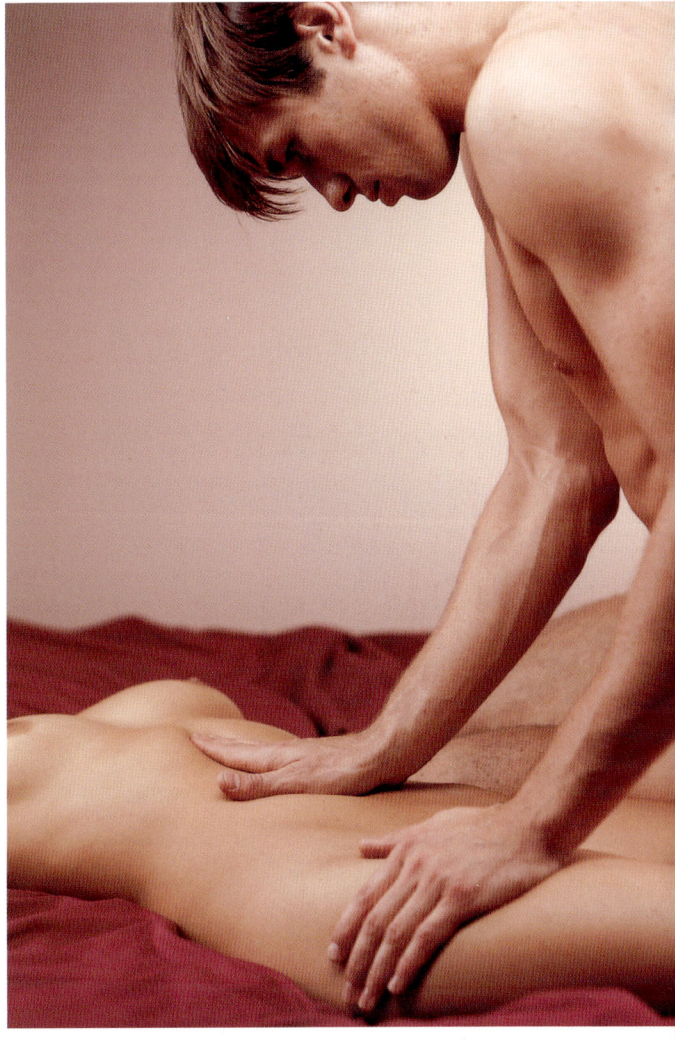

Continue rotating your hand and, when you have completed about a quarter of a circle, gradually turn your hand over onto its palm as you rotate, bringing your elbow level with the bed or floor. Ensure that the supporting hand remains passive, giving a sense of secure comfort.

With your palm down, continue rotating the hand in a clockwise direction. Now turn your hand over so that the palm is once again facing upward by the time the circle is completed. Your forearm should be upright, with the elbow directly above the hand. Throughout the sequence the hand should travel clockwise in a gentle flow – this will soon become easy. Repeat these three steps 12 times. As a finishing touch, rest your palm lightly over the navel, allowing your hand to rise and fall very slightly with each breath.

Inner thighs

Women tend to find the inner thigh a more sensitive area than men. A light caressing touch close to the vulva is almost as suggestive as a direct touch itself might be. Men seem to prefer a caress that actually lightly touches or brushes on the penis. Either way, in this part of the massage you finally build up to genital contact. With your partner still lying on her back, position yourself at your partner's side, at mid-thigh level. As this is a highly erotic and sensitive area, be extra careful with your first touch.

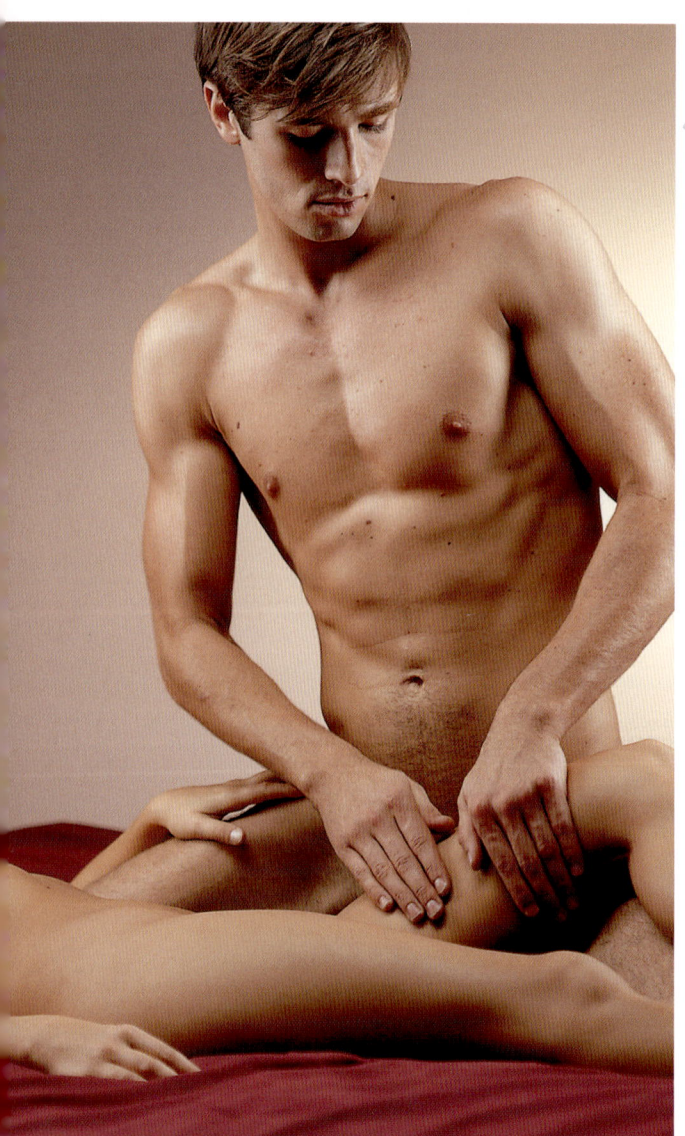

1 With your hands placed on your partner's inner thigh at the level of the top of the knee, stroke one hand after the other as you gradually work upward, then lightly brush the genitals before descending in smoothing strokes back to the knee area. Repeat a few times, nonchalantly going about your strokes as if impropriety were not in any way part of your intention! Be sure to incorporate the back of the knee as you move up and down the leg.

Eroticism and the genitals

Whatever technique you choose to use on the genitals, the goal should not be mere arousal. Given the setting and the attraction between you, arousal is an inevitable consequence of loving touch, but don't compartmentalize the genitals, focusing on them with arousal as your main purpose. Instead, look to connect them to the rest of the body. When you successfully do that you demonstrate to your partner that you see her sexual organs as more than just objects to pleasure you, but as part of a whole person and personality. Arguably this is the definition of, and difference between, pornography and eroticism.

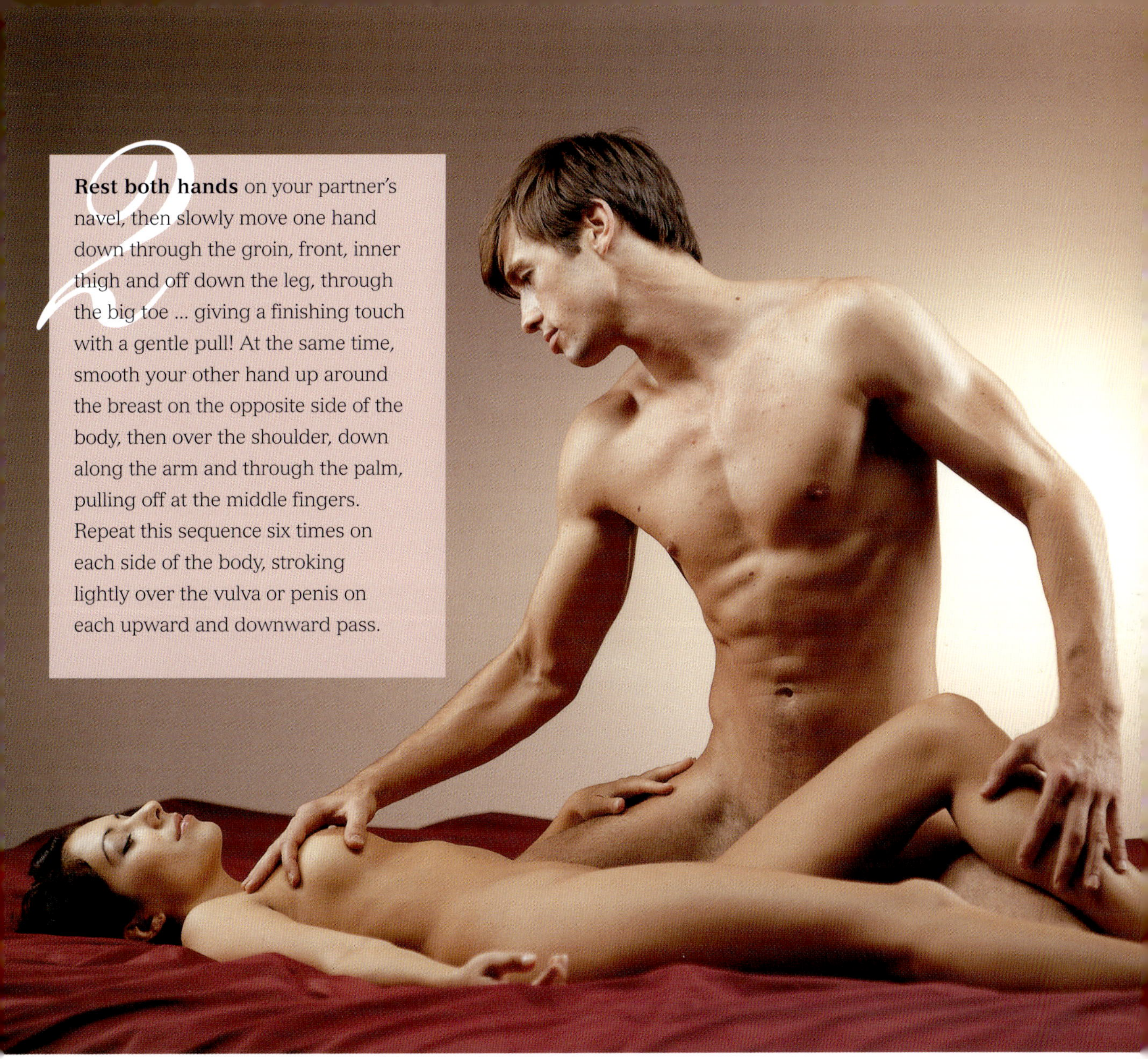

Rest both hands on your partner's navel, then slowly move one hand down through the groin, front, inner thigh and off down the leg, through the big toe ... giving a finishing touch with a gentle pull! At the same time, smooth your other hand up around the breast on the opposite side of the body, then over the shoulder, down along the arm and through the palm, pulling off at the middle fingers. Repeat this sequence six times on each side of the body, stroking lightly over the vulva or penis on each upward and downward pass.

Trace the outline of the genitals with a single finger, as if sketching a chalk outline. Work gently over and around the area with tiny circles of fingers or tongue and lips. Kiss one set of lips while you fondle another, suck a finger as you lightly grip its larger twin. Look to enact on a non-genital area your intention for its genital counterpart. Suck, kiss and caress a less obvious reflection of mountain or valley. Remember, the most sensitive organ of the body is the brain and the most erotic technique is imagination.

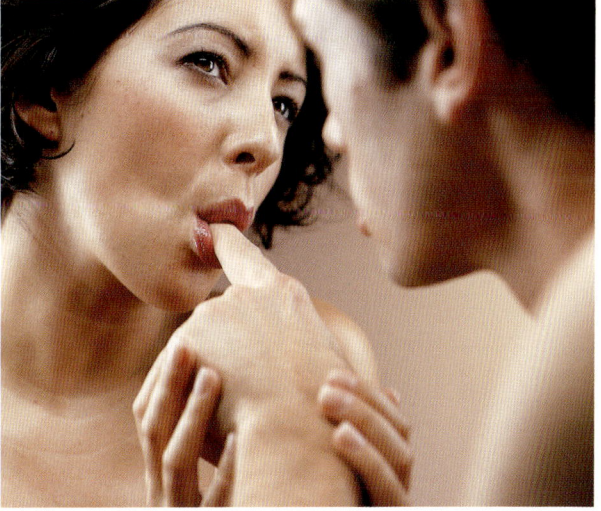

The feet

For some, this extra-sensitive pleasure zone is too ticklish to be pleasurable. The best advice is to start as you mean to go on – be firm with your technique and persevere. As a prelude (especially appropriate if you are using these steps for a "quickie" foot massage), wash and dry your partner's feet and massage in some stimulating foot lotion. Ask your partner to turn over and lie face down on the massage surface, and position yourself in front of the feet or sitting lightly on the thighs.

Kneading Using both thumbs, knead into the soft areas of the sole of one foot, rubbing back and forth or in small circular movements, ensuring that you're supporting the foot with your other fingers.

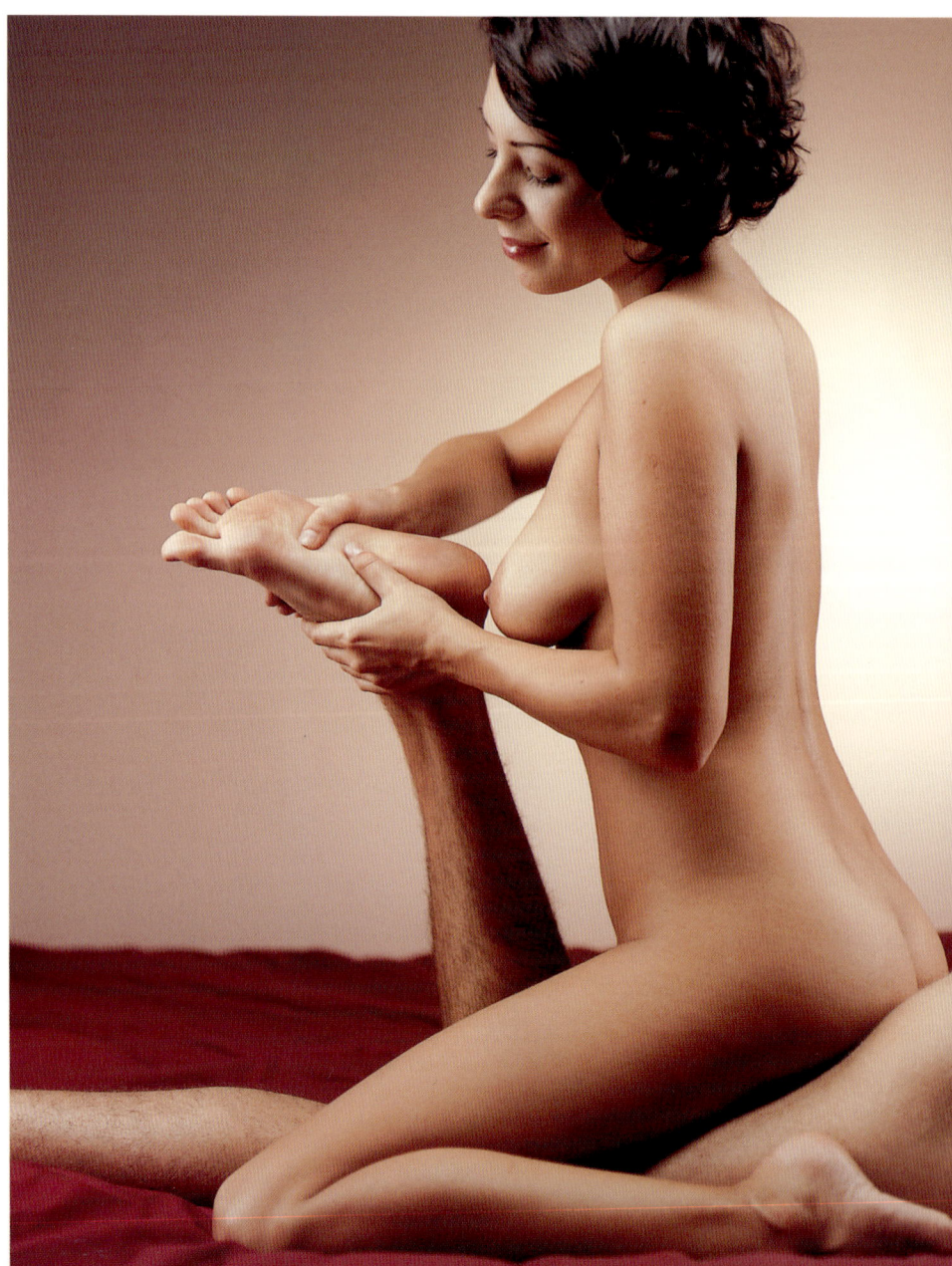

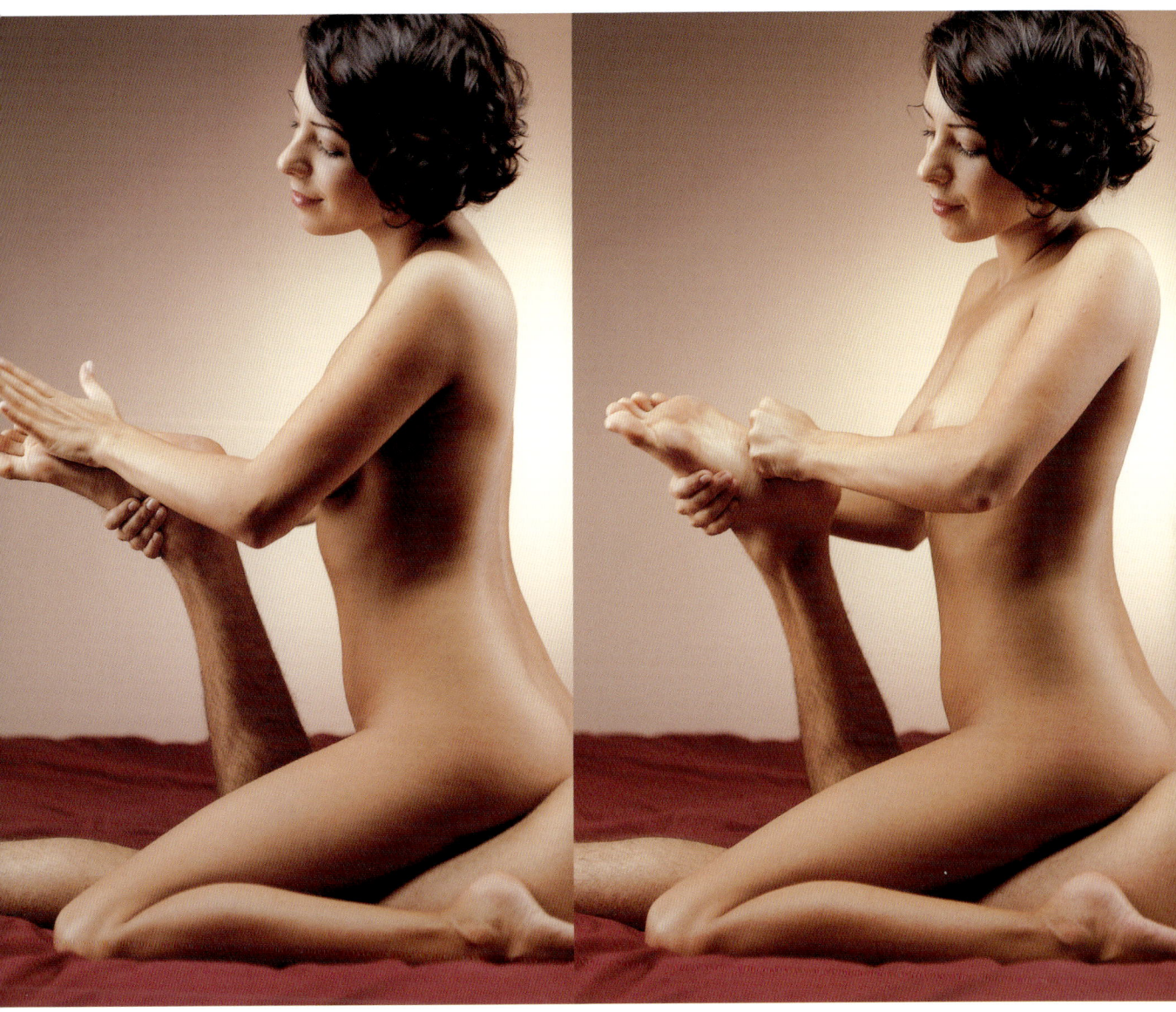

Arch friction Begin to apply firmer pressure with the same strokes. Supporting the foot underneath, concentrate the pressure through your fingers, stroking into the arch of the foot. You can even allow a long stroke that includes the forearm and elbow.

Knuckling Circle with the flat part of your knuckles around the arch and up into the heel using firm pressure. Combine circling with forward and backward movements. This is ideal for warming cold and stiff feet. Repeat the sequence on the other foot.

Up to the buttocks

This section of the massage sequence can release lots of tension in the legs, leaving your partner feeling lighter and much more relaxed as a result. He should be lying face down on the massage surface, with you positioned beside his feet.

1 Stroke upward from the ankle to the back of the knee, using either the back of the hand or the middle finger. Stroke around the center of the back of the knee in a clockwise direction with your middle finger. (For this stroke, support the leg with your free hand at the shin.) Repeat on the other leg.

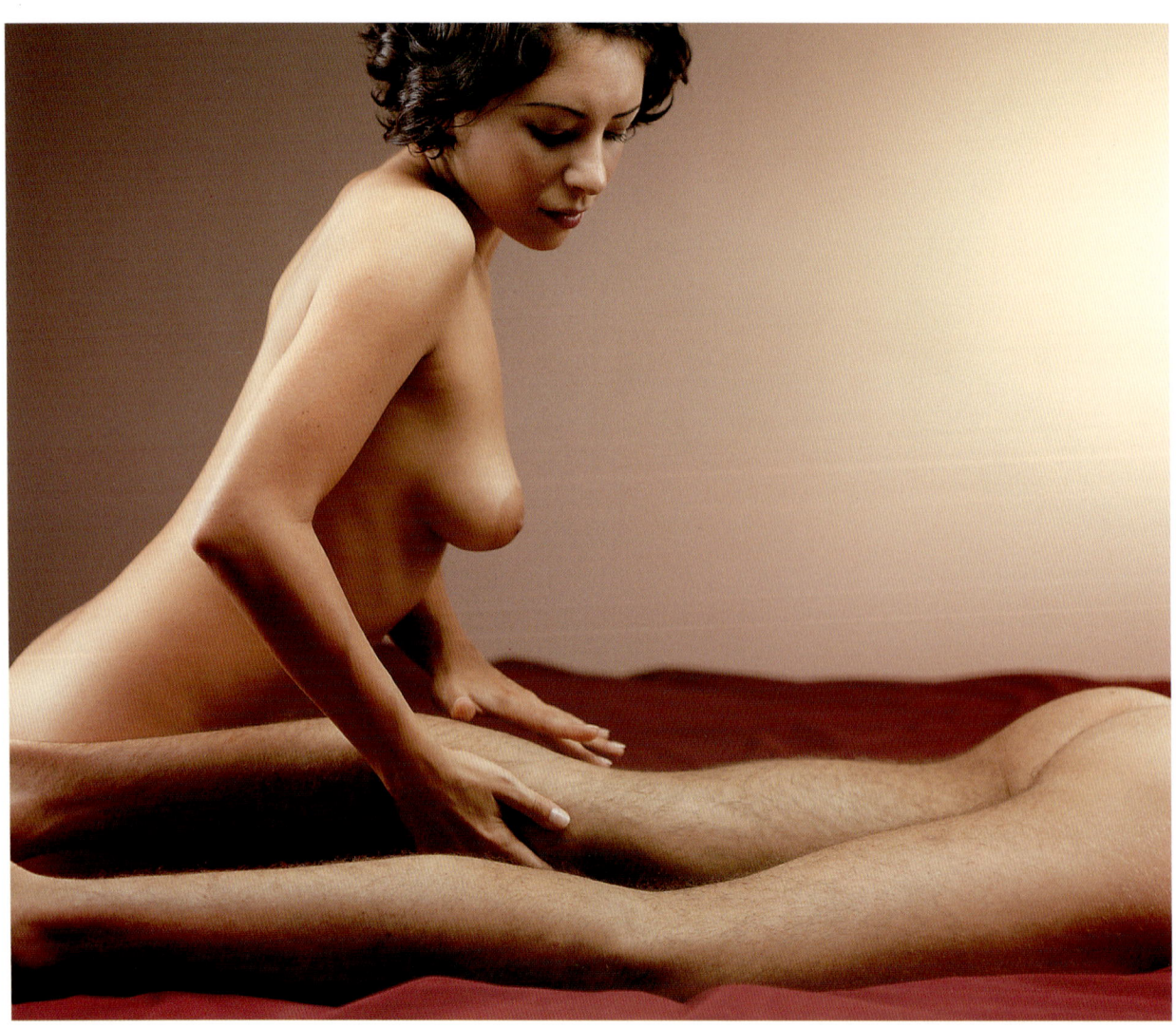

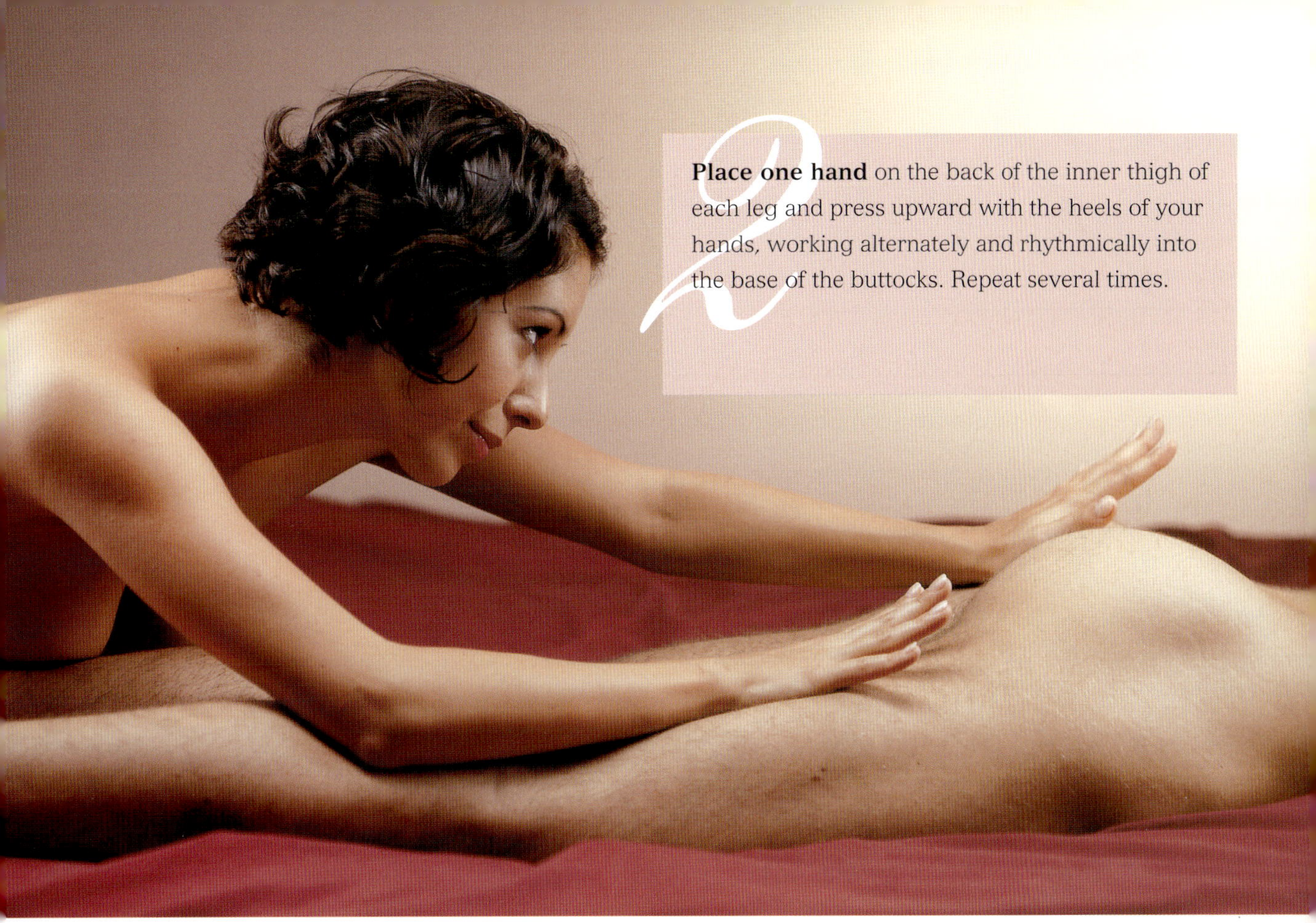

Place one hand on the back of the inner thigh of each leg and press upward with the heels of your hands, working alternately and rhythmically into the base of the buttocks. Repeat several times.

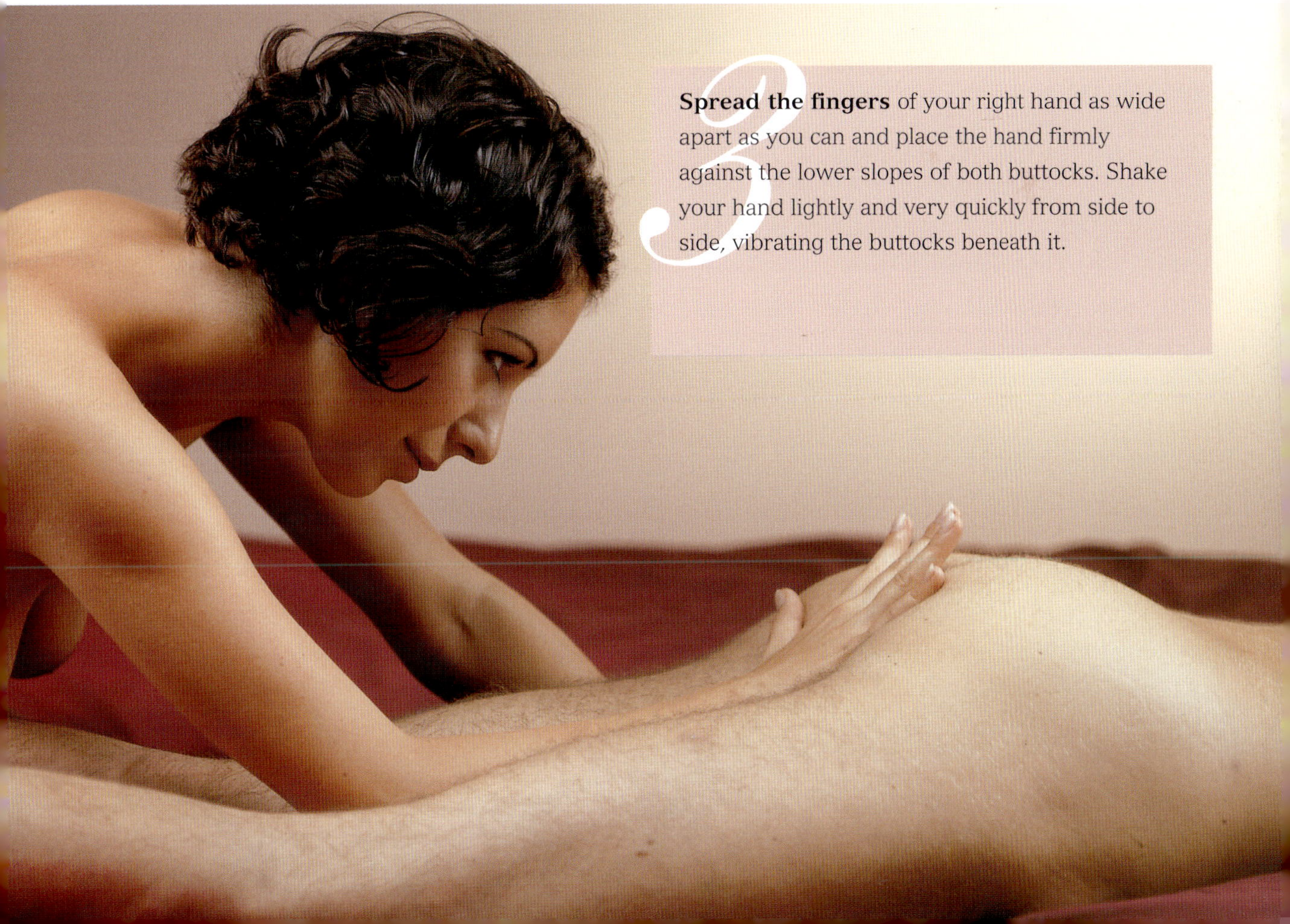

Spread the fingers of your right hand as wide apart as you can and place the hand firmly against the lower slopes of both buttocks. Shake your hand lightly and very quickly from side to side, vibrating the buttocks beneath it.

The lower back

The lower back, base of the spine and coccyx (tailbone) are the sites of two psychic centers, the muladhara and svadhisthana chakras (wheels of energy). Within two fingerwidths of one another, they are the root and abode of Kundalini Shakti (female serpent energy) and the sexual center that disseminates the most powerful of divine energies. Arousal and conscious management of this energy is the goal and secret of Tantric sex.

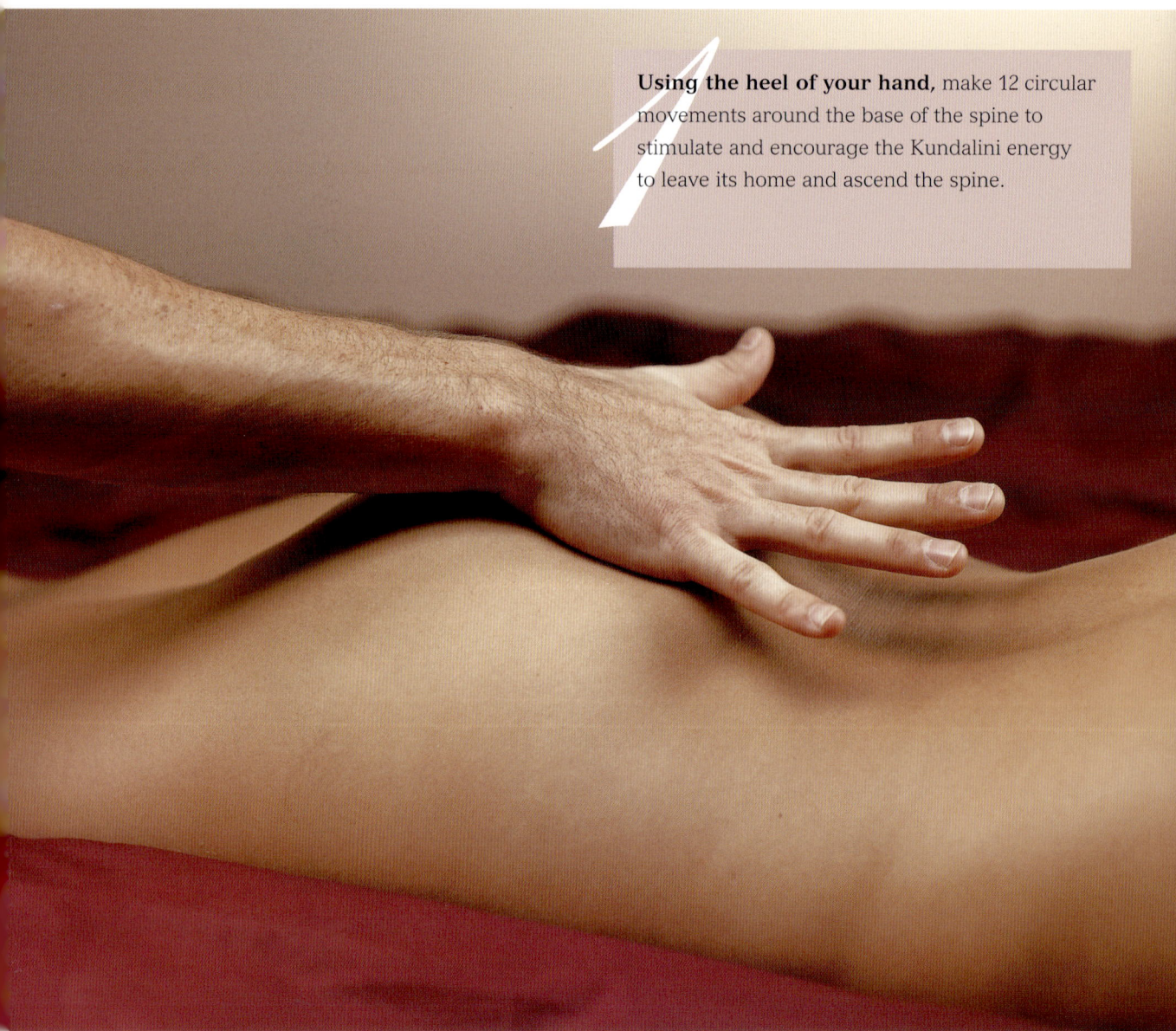

1 Using the heel of your hand, make 12 circular movements around the base of the spine to stimulate and encourage the Kundalini energy to leave its home and ascend the spine.

Begin fan stroking on the lower back – position your hands on either side of the base of the spine, then glide them up, molding them to the shape of the hips and waist with a light touch before leaning into the hands for firm, even pressure as you glide them along the sides of the rib cage then in toward the spine. With your thumbs on either side of the spine, work down the back to the starting position and repeat several times. Allow your hands to flow in smooth circles.

Hot tip
Circle the base vertebra with the tip of the middle finger in a clockwise direction, then rest your palm on the area to heat it up. Hold for four to five breaths, then remove your warming hand.

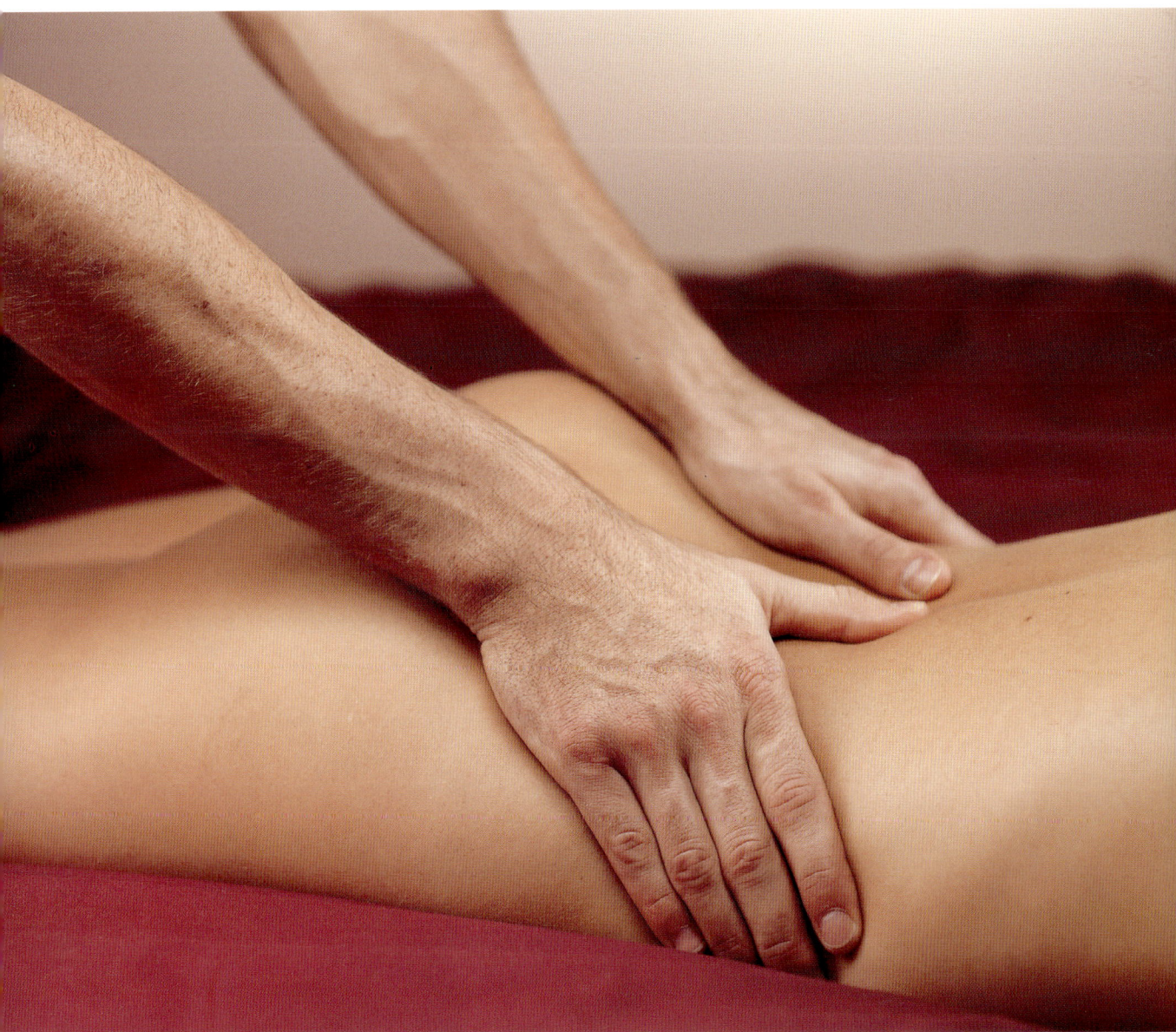

The lower back

Infinity ribbon

This figure eight technique is a bold, reassuring stroke. Throughout this sequence, one hand should be placed over the other, with the fingers on the top hand sitting between those of the lower hand. Using both hands allows for variations of strong and light strokes and the "guiding" upper hand disguises any uncertain movements. For this part of the massage, sit on your partner's left side at hip level.

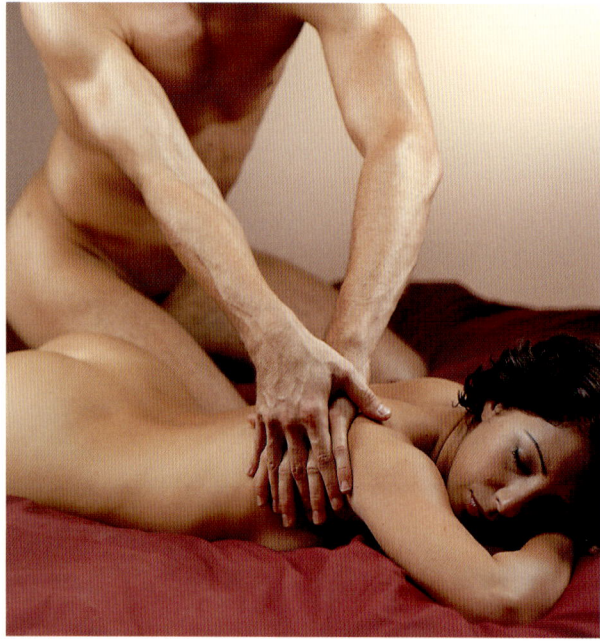 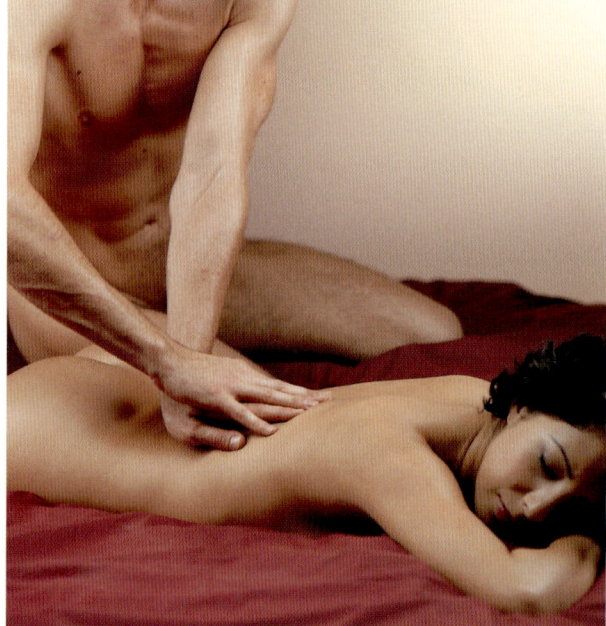

1 Position your hands on the right side of the body, just below the armpit, then slide them up over the right shoulder, lightly hooking the hands over the shoulder muscles. Glide the hands diagonally across the spine and under the left shoulder blade. Work your hands around the left side of the torso, up onto the left shoulder, then diagonally across the spine again to the right side of the body and back round to the starting position. Your hands have traced a figure eight pattern – an infinity ribbon – on your partner's back. Repeat this gliding motion and feel the shoulder muscles relax beneath your touch.

2 Continue the stroke seamlessly as you work down the back. Make sure you don't apply pressure to the spine itself and remember that relaxation comes from multiple caresses. Keep constant contact, being aware of the rhythmic flow of the continuous movements.

Hot tip
The buttocks hold a lot of tension and respond well to this technique. Move from a stronger to a lighter stroke, even teasing the buttock crease.

Pleasure zones

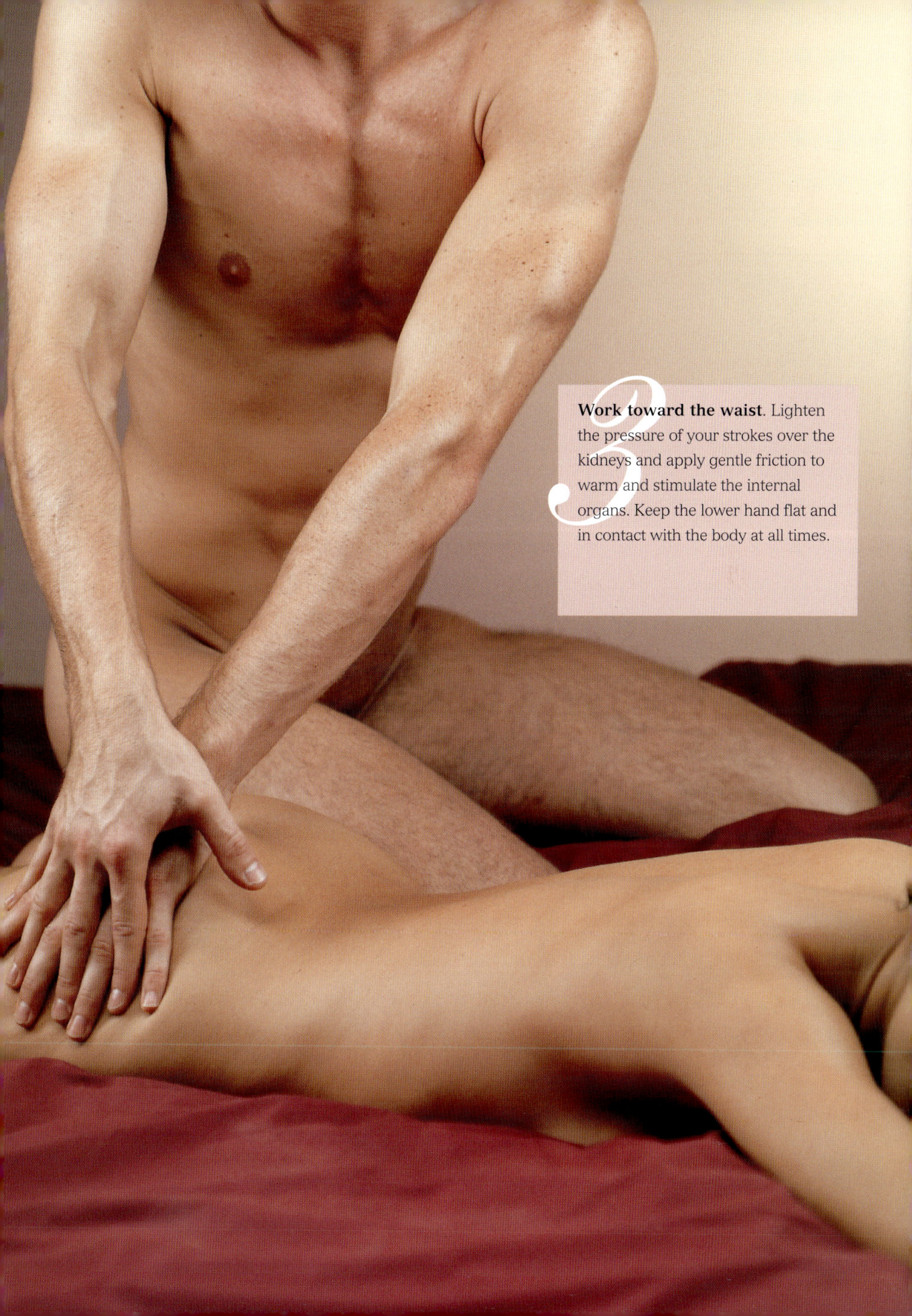

3 Work toward the waist. Lighten the pressure of your strokes over the kidneys and apply gentle friction to warm and stimulate the internal organs. Keep the lower hand flat and in contact with the body at all times.

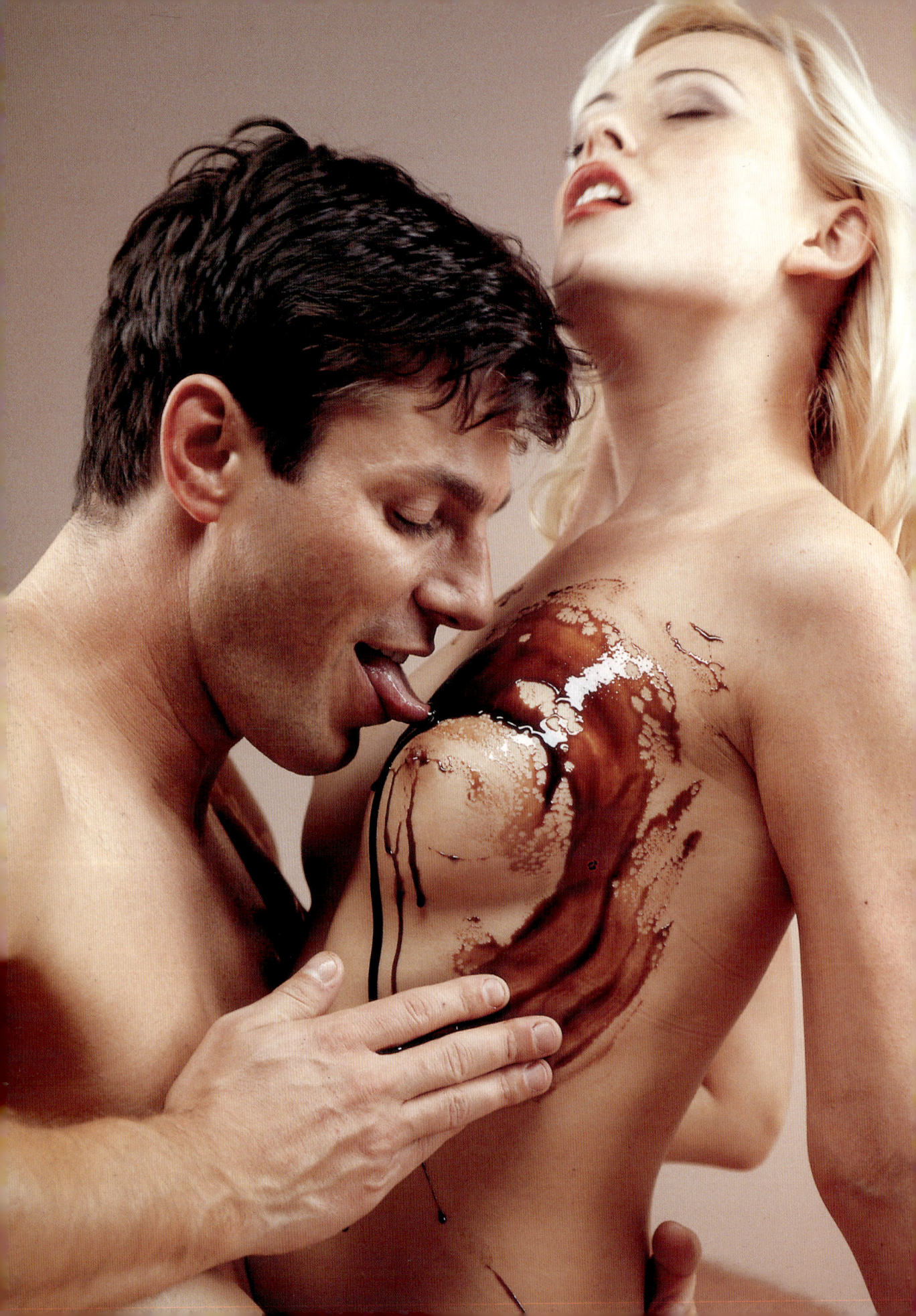

Teasing & tantalizing

Experiment with blindfolds, silk, fire and ice, feathers and chocolate. Discover a multitude of novel skin sensations.

Fabulous feathers

From the ancient Egyptians to the Hopi tribe today, feathers have long been used as an aid to massage and healing. They are imbued with symbolism, conjuring up feelings of lightness and freedom, and are especially helpful for unlocking tense muscles and releasing inhibitions.

Sensual, luxurious feathers can greatly enhance an erotic massage. Try using a variety, from downy mini feathers to silky ostrich plumes, stick-mounted ticklers and fluffy boas. Remember that too light a touch may be unbearably ticklish and could spoil the flow, especially in vulnerable places such as under the arms or along the side of the rib cage. It is usually best to start with the buttocks using long slow strokes and medium pressure, and then continue with small, light circles as excitement builds. Let your partner luxuriate in the gentlest of touches and be alert to reactions; does he strain away from the sensation or relax into it? As always, don't rush on to the next area until you are sure your partner is ready. Move around the body, varying the way you use the feathers – try long, lingering strokes up and down the spine and little caresses that tease the erogenous zones such as his neck and belly.

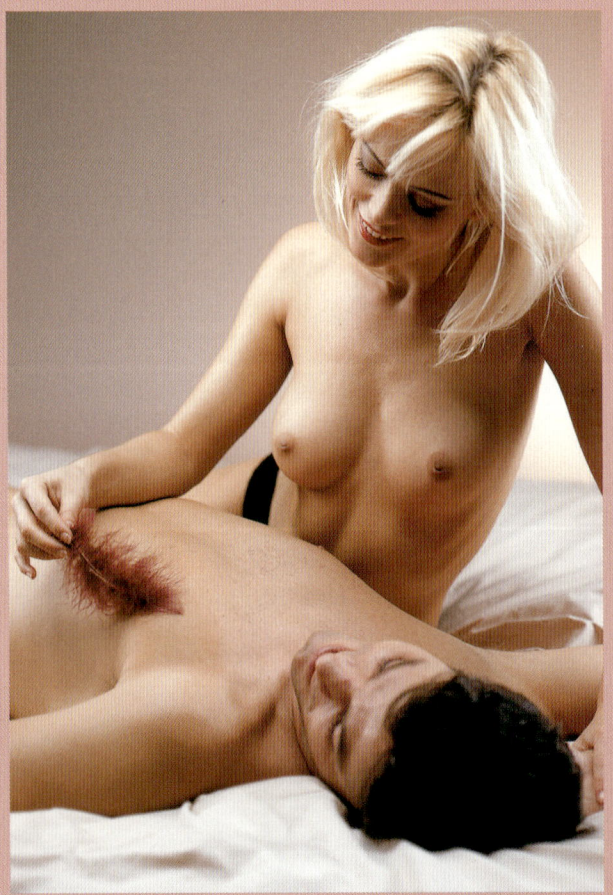

lingering strokes up and down the spine and little **caresses** that **tease** the **erogenous** zones

Hot tip
The most intense and exquisite sensations come from long strokes that tease the contours of the body and trace a cleft between muscle groups or along the ridge of a muscle. Apart from obvious areas such as the neck, shoulders and back, try the biceps and forearms, inner thighs and calves. Avoid feet and toes, and especially ticklish areas inside the upper arms, armpits and sides of the torso.

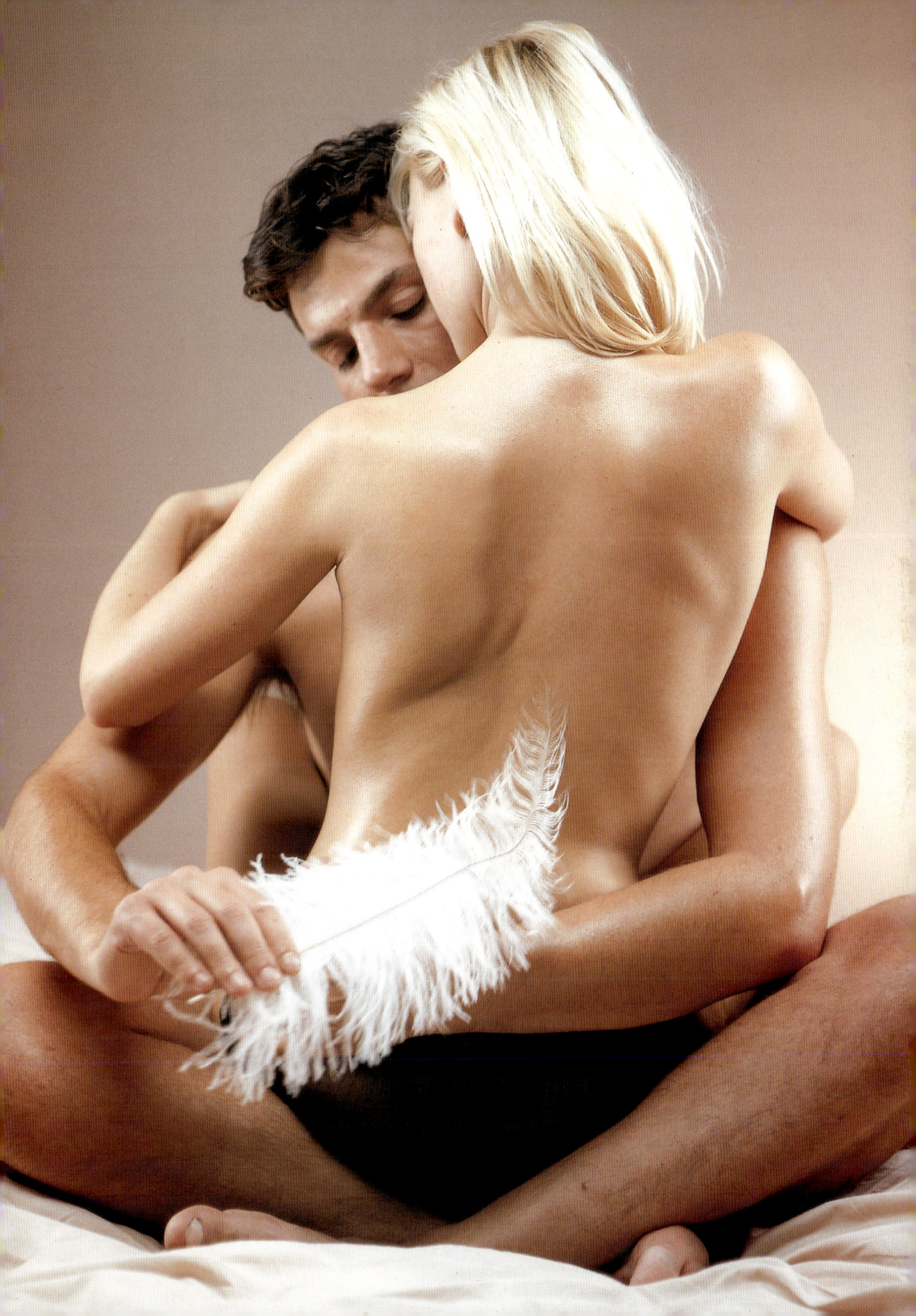

Smooth and silky

Silk gloves give a whole new meaning to back massage. They eliminate the need for oils and lotions and give instant, highly charged results with very little prior preparation.

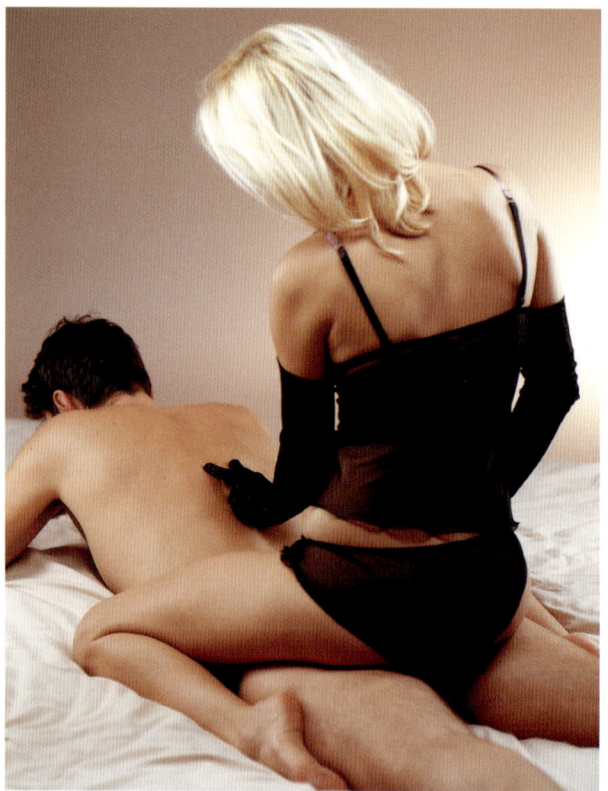 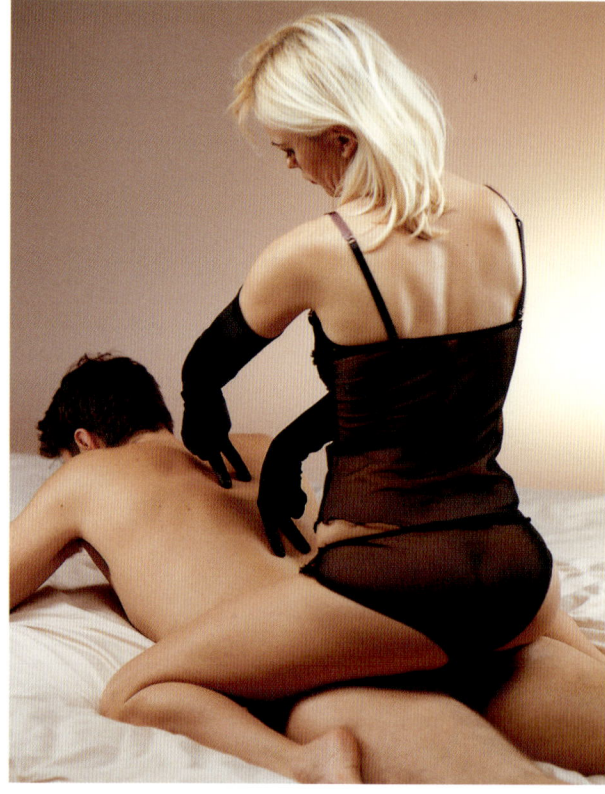

1 Tracing and trailing This is a technique that is much more subtle than it looks. Make a "V" shape with your index and middle fingers, curling the other fingers into the palm with the aid of the thumb. Place your fingers on either side of the vertebrae at the nape of the neck and trace down along the muscles on either side of the spine very gently, molding your fingers to the shape of each vertebra in turn. End with a circle around the base vertebra (tailbone). Now trail the backs of the fingers up along the edges of the spine, then repeat this step.

2 Double trace Make "V"s with both hands. With the right hand, work down the back as before, but only a little way, then lift your hand off the body and begin to follow the path of your right hand down the back with the left hand, starting a little farther down the back this time. Keep your hands flowing down the back one after another, never losing contact with your partner's skin by having at least one hand touching it at all times. Each time you start a stroke, begin a little farther down the back and, in this way, gradually work your way down to the base. Now trail the backs of the fingers up to the starting position. Repeat this series of strokes six times. This technique creates a "wave" of pleasure down the back.

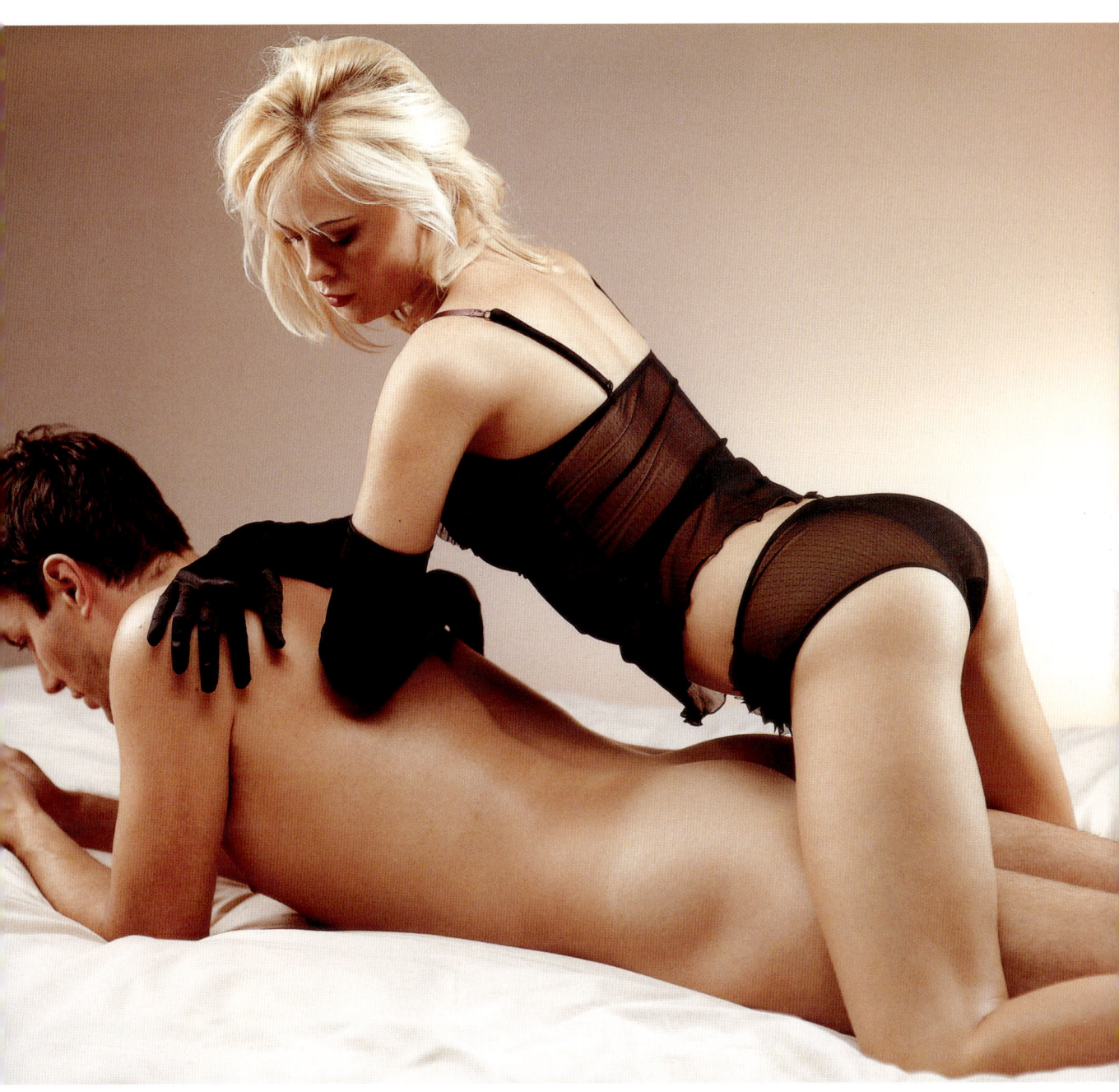

Forearm press Place the forearms together on the middle of your partner's back, hands molding around the sides. Slowly press down on his back and spread your forearms apart, stretching the skin beneath. Keep your arms moving at the same pace and pressure as each other until one forearm reaches the top of the back and the other crosses over the buttocks. Then lift the forearms off the skin to return to the starting position. Repeat this move six times.

Hot tip
Whether you are wearing silk underwear or sensual lingerie, massage all over your partner's body with all of your body, then take off your clothing and trail it all over the pleasure zones.

Hair play

One of the reasons why many of us love going to the hairdresser is that we adore having people play with our hair. Hair play can be charged with eroticism and, as another form of sensual touch, is a playful addition to your seductive massage.

Running your fingers through one another's hair (or across the scalp), stroking, pulling and rubbing can be very satisfying. If you have long hair, use it to tease and tantalize your partner's pleasure zones with long, streamlined strokes or short, sharp, whipping ones. No doubt your partner enjoys the way your hair looks, so allow him to enjoy how it feels, too. If you don't have long hair, re-create the sensation with a soft tassel. If your partner has long hair, why not make the most of it? As your fingers become tangled in his or her hair, enjoy the feel of the long locks, be they smooth and silky or luxuriously wavy. Your pleasure is enhanced by the knowledge that your touch is giving your partner wonderful sensations at the same time.

Hot tip
Wrap a warm towel around your partner's head and twist the fabric into a topknot. Hold the base of the neck and the topknot and gently stretch the neck to ease out tension.

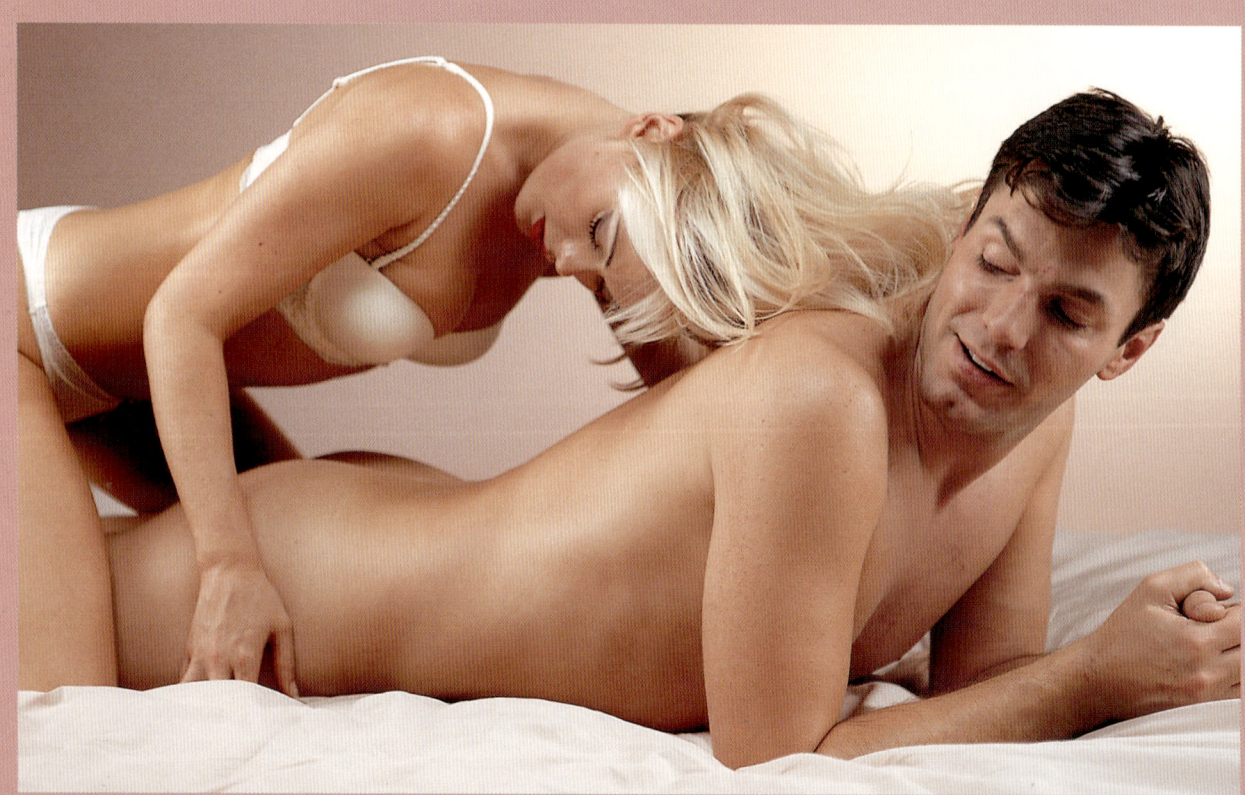

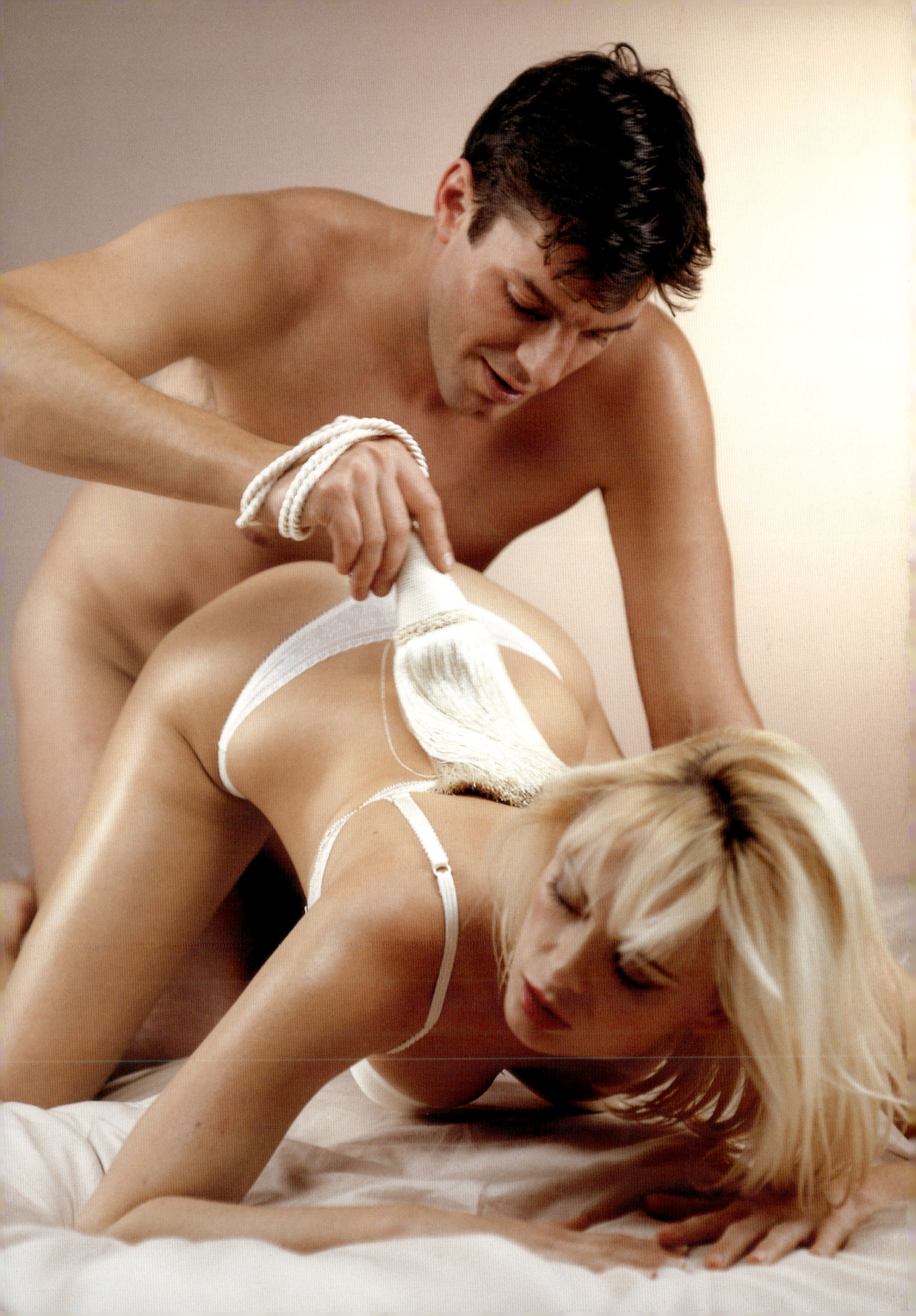

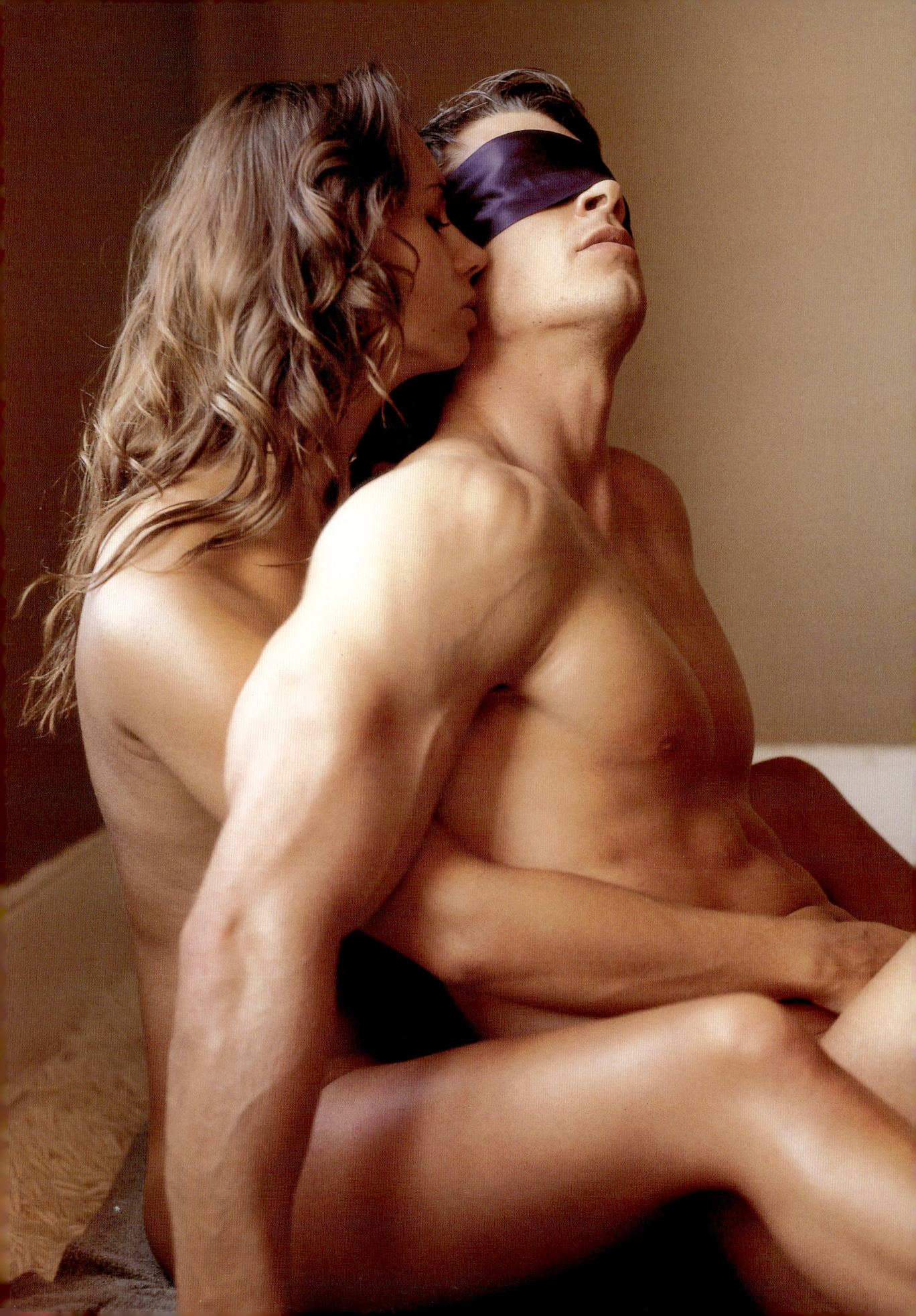

Using playful touch

An element of sex play can be introduced to erotic touch to further turn up the heat. Power games bring another level of eroticism to the massage, moving away from innocence to a feeling of delicious wickedness!

Blindfold sensations

It is generally acknowledged that when one sense is curtailed, all the other senses are heightened. The simplest blindfold, whether a man's tie or the belt from a woman's robe, is quite effective. For a subtler suggestion why not use a pair of hose (silk or nylon) that has been worn earlier and is infused with a mixture of body pheromones and a favorite scent. Legend tells that Casanova, the great lover, used to wear a handkerchief around his testicles to pick up his natural secretions!

Blindfolding might make your partner a little anxious (and excited). He won't know what will happen, or from where sensation will come. For some who are truly concerned or alarmed, make sure those first surprises are gentle ones – a loving touch, a sensuous kiss, the lightest caress with a feather.

It is surprising how difficult it is to imagine what is making such a thrilling and unusual sensation on the body when you are being touched while blindfolded. Improvise with a pastry wheel, a meat tenderizer, a spatula – in fact anything with knobbled or serrated surfaces and edges. Even forks, spoons and assorted cutlery (either cold or warmed) can surprise and startle. You can smack, prod, poke, smooth, titillate, tickle and slap. Your partner will be sure to give you clues if you read his responses well. Encourage him to vocalize his feelings and you can pleasure or "punish" by fulfilling or withdrawing certain pleasures. Experimentation can be fun, will empower the giver and sensitize even the most jaded sexual palette.

Although the blindfold scenario is more commonly enacted by one partner on another, you could trade roles or, if it is safe and you're well organized, you could both be blindfolded. The only thing is, will either of you cheat?

Fire and ice

Heightened sensations while blindfolded would not be complete without "fire and ice" treatment. Using an ice cube, trace round the aureole of the nipple (male or female) for outstanding results. Is this a case of being cruel to be kind? Well, yes. The natural warmth of lips is a strong enough contrast to the ice to introduce the opposites of heat and cold. Alternatively use an item that has been left near a heater to warm. (Be sure to test it on your own inner arm first so you don't risk burning your beloved.) Contrasting applications on various parts of the body, especially the genitals, provide an exquisite "torture."

Tie me up – tie me down

If you wish to take things further, consider tying your partner to a bedpost, sofa or any other object. The knot or restraining device does not have to be truly restrictive – ask your partner to choose how tight or strong it should be. Don't be alarmed if his or her tastes run to a rather more severe level than you would like or have imagined. Everyone has different tolerance levels. Your partner should have a "safe" word (see page 12) to use if things get out of hand, so go with the flow and let your imagination craft a sexy scene. This is one role-playing scenario where you can both let your imaginations run wild within ultimately safe confines – the essence of erotic!

Hot chocolate kisses

Sex and chocolate are synonymous. Every chocolate advertisement worth watching has sexy connotations. So use chocolate to paint hot messages on your partner, polish them off with your tongue and finish with a hot chocolate kiss.

Breaking the rules
From a very young age we are taught that it is "naughty" to make a mess with food – this is essential discipline with a messy toddler! And being "naughty" – doing things you are not supposed to do to break convention and boundaries – is an erotic trigger.

Sweet indulgence
Being in itself a sybaritic luxury, chocolate is the ideal accompaniment to the ideas below. These suggestions are minor transgressions, and if chocolate doesn't appeal, they can be allied with any opulent and sensual food – crushed or pulped soft fruits such as peaches, strawberries and even avocado are perfect. Whatever you choose, it should be a taste you enjoy and associate with indulgence. Other sweet treats might include honey, cream, custard or yogurt. Remember – there is not a food that exists that is not enhanced by the scent and texture of a human body.

Getting creative
Ideas for application can vary from dripping and smearing to painting on with a paintbrush or basting brush. You can try spelling out a word – perhaps a name, or something rude or provocative – on your partner's flesh and ask her to guess what that word is. Try smearing on the chocolate with your bare hands, making both of you "dirty." And of course, licking or kissing is the natural way to deal with the resultant mess.

> use **chocolate** to paint hot messages on your partner, **polish** them off with your **tongue** and finish with a **hot** chocolate kiss

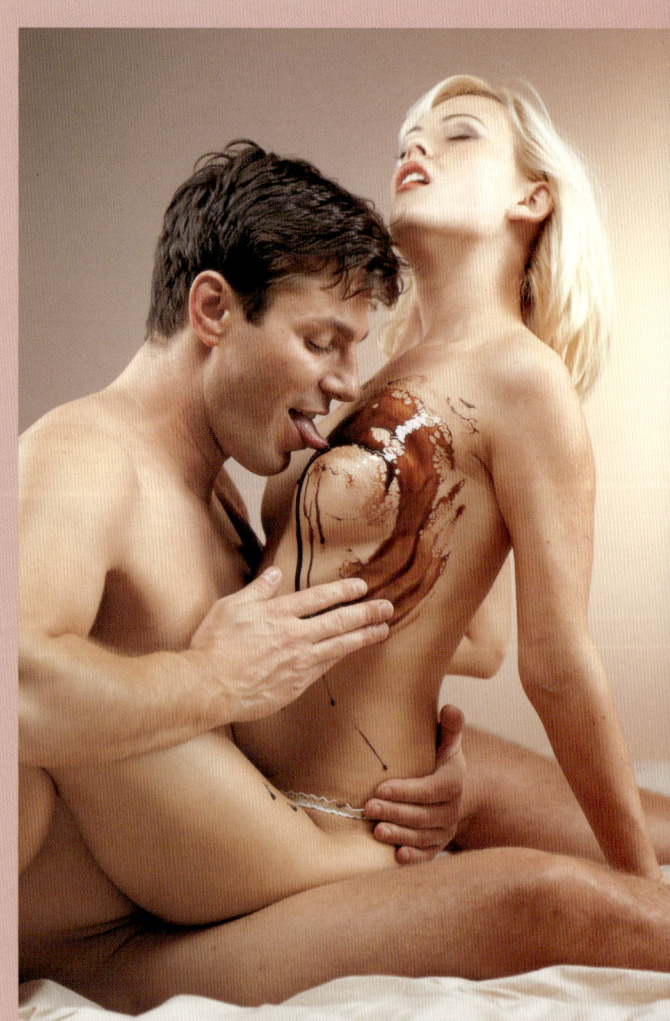

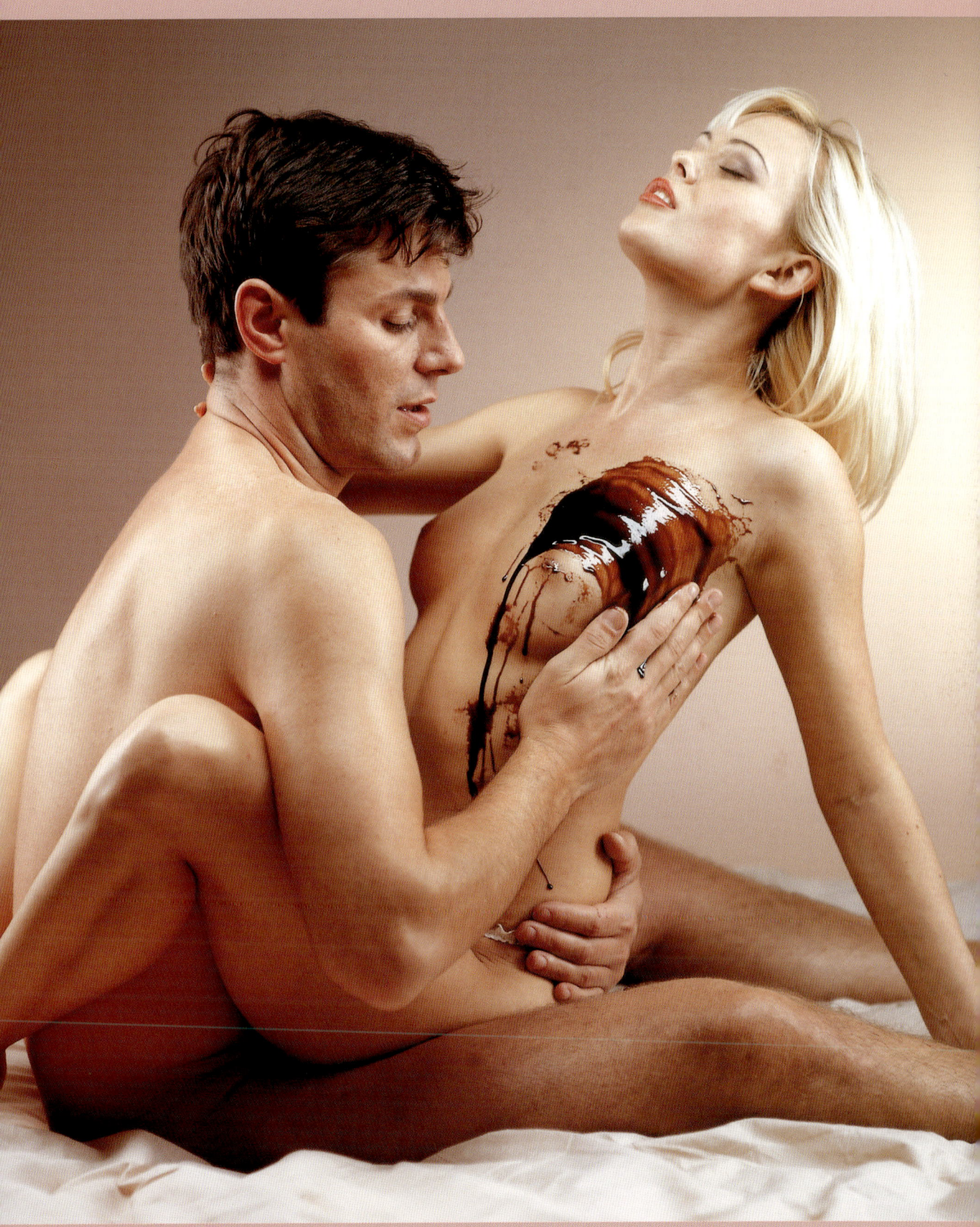

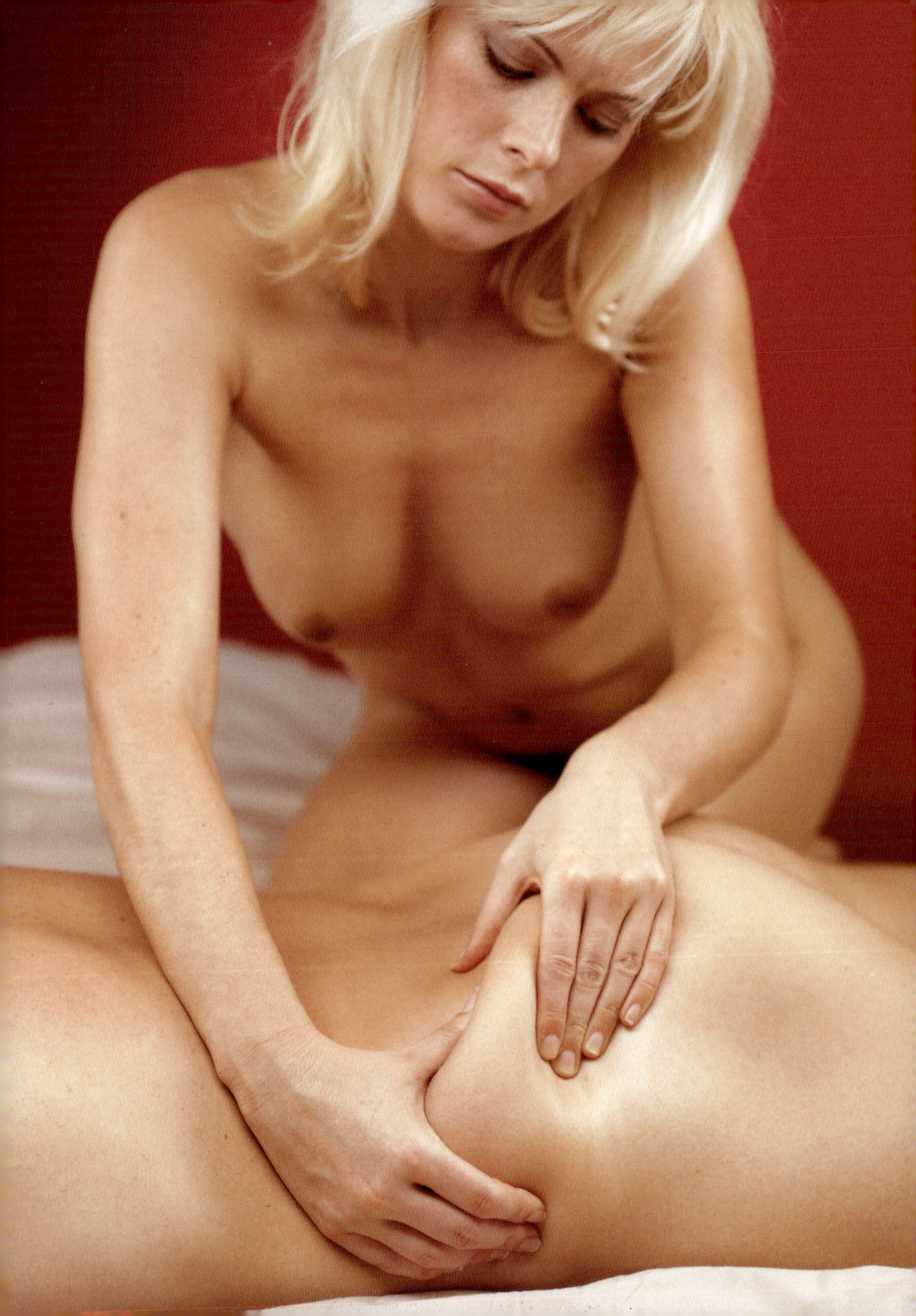

Stimulating & arousing

Try out invigorating techniques such as percussion, edging, squeezing, cupping and kneading.

Before you begin

This section of massage techniques, to be performed in the sequence in which they appear, is designed to stimulate and arouse a sluggish system and tired body. (However, any of the techniques may be used to augment a customized massage program you put together with the aid of this book.) If you or your partner feels unfit or run down – either physically or emotionally – this massage will help to give you a boost.

There are quite a few friction movements in this sequence, so you'll need to use a massage medium. If you elect to use oil rather than talc or a premixed lotion, consider blending it with the mixes of essential oils given below. These are known to stimulate a torpid physique, revive a jaded emotional palate and revitalize a lethargic mental attitude. When using essential oils it is advisable not to use your best sheets as they might get stained. Protect your sheets with a large, warmed bath towel, which also adds an extra level of comfort for you and your partner.

Positioning your partner

Ask your partner to lie on his or her front, with legs relaxed from the hips to the toes, feet in line with the hips and heels dropped outward slightly. In most situations you will need to place a large cushion or pillow beneath the chest to allow the neck to relax forward without strain. Your partner's head should be resting lightly on the forehead or be turned 90° to either side. Position the arms either alongside and a little away from the torso, or so that they are raised above shoulder level with one hand on the back of the other beneath the forehead. Depending on how long and vigorous the massage is, the prone position may need to be slightly adjusted to ensure maximum comfort. From time to time check that your partner is comfortable, adding or adjusting cushions or pillows as necessary. Remember to ensure that there are no drafts in the room and that the temperature is to your partner's liking.

Enlivening essential oil blends

Invigorating and stimulating
This blend also helps to boost poor circulation: basil oil (two drops), patchouli oil (two drops), juniper or rosemary oil (two drops) mixed with two teaspoons of a carrier oil. Caution: do not use on anyone suffering from high blood pressure.

Revitalizing
Ideal for easing aches, pains and tired muscles, regulating menstruation and alleviating water retention: eucalyptus oil (two drops), rosemary oil (two drops), sage oil (one drop) mixed with two teaspoons of carrier oil. Caution: do not use on anyone suffering from high blood pressure.

stimulate a sluggish body, **revive** a jaded emotional state and **revitalize** a lethargic mental attitude

Stimulating & arousing

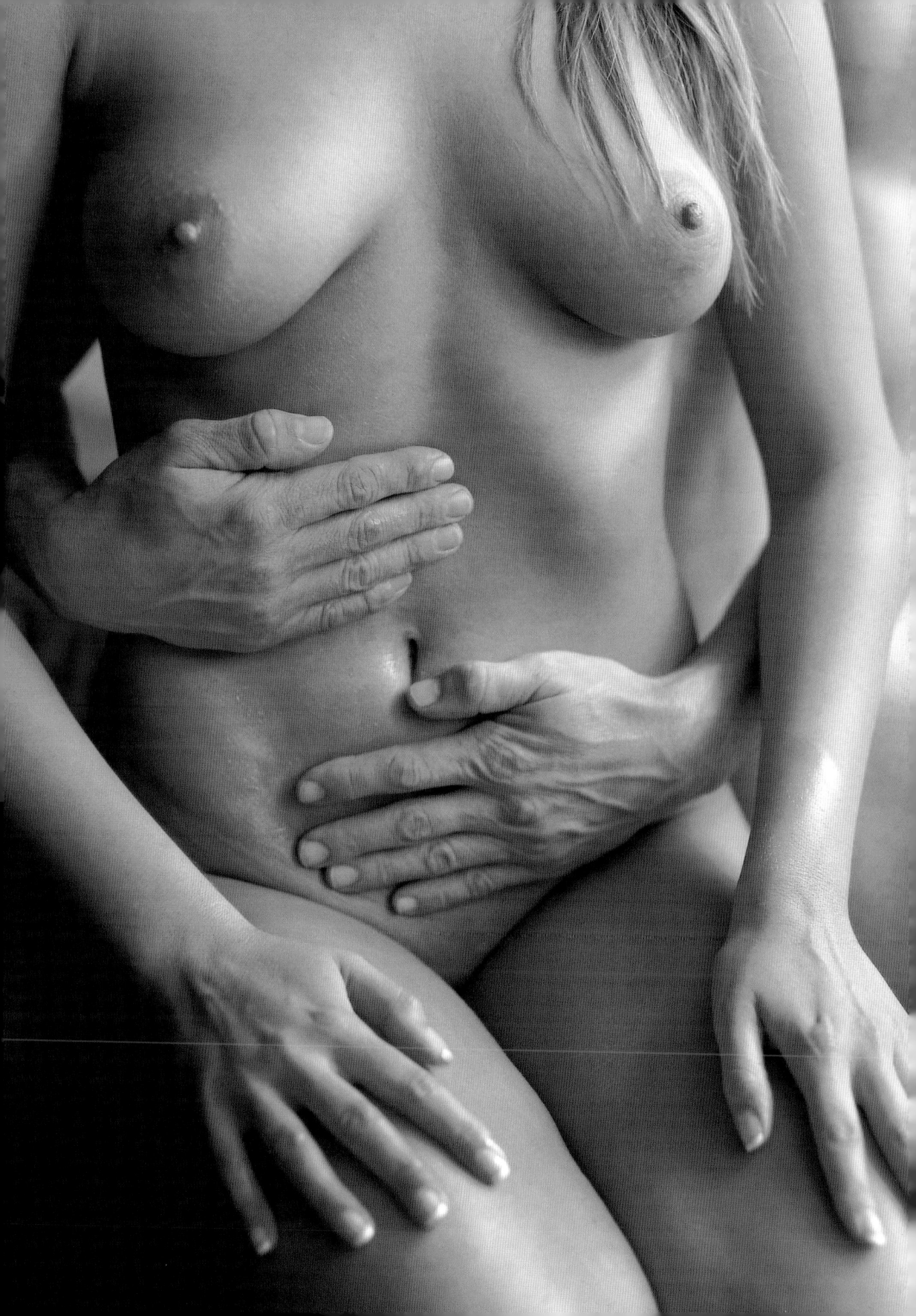

Beginning the massage

This series of strokes provides the perfect start to an invigorating massage by warming the muscles. Make sure your partner is comfortable on his front, then sit astride the hips with his buttocks nestled between your upper thighs.

1 Warming up This technique can be used on all parts of the body to begin and end a massage and as a transitional stroke to ease from one movement to another. It is also used to oil or lubricate the whole torso in preparation for a range of massage strokes. Use the entire flat of both hands working in unison to make soothing strokes. Experiment with different speeds, pressures and rhythms, always looking for feedback – vocal and non-vocal. Long, fluent strokes will limber you up and make you aware of your potential range of movements – you might find you need to adjust your position to reach all areas of the body without strain. They will also warm the muscle groups for what is to come.

2 Fir tree Place both hands on the lower back on either side of the spine with the thumb and index finger of each hand about 1½ inches apart and hands close together to form a fir-tree shape. Using the whole of both hands and maintaining the fir-tree shape, smooth up along the edges of the spine, then part your hands to cup them over the tops of the shoulders and glide down the outer edges of the shoulder blades to the sides of the body. In a continuous and fluid motion, draw the hands down either side of the body to return to the starting position. Repeat this technique six times and, as an alternative, sit at your partner's head and reverse the procedure, from neck to base. To fine-tune, exhale in unison on the upward strokes and inhale on the downward strokes.

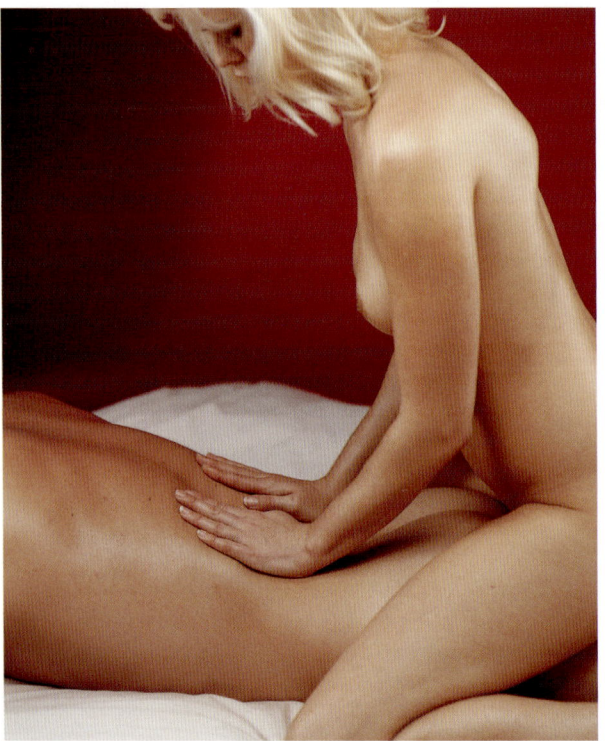
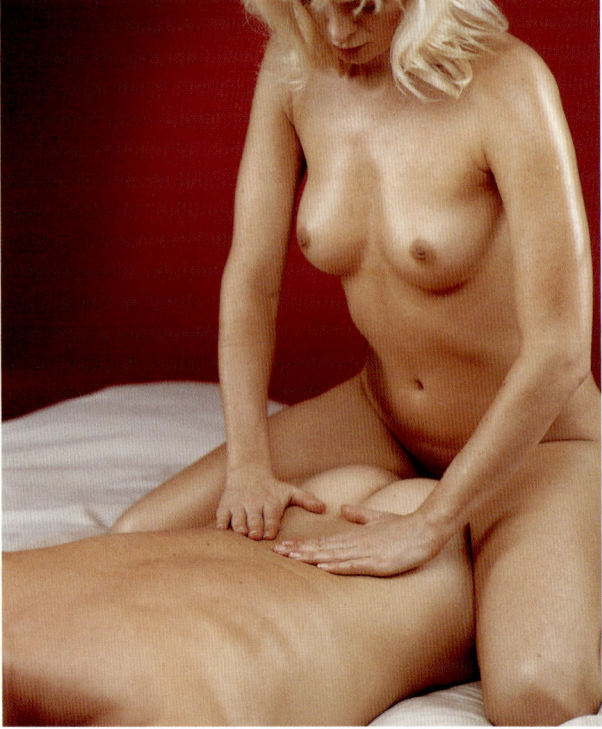

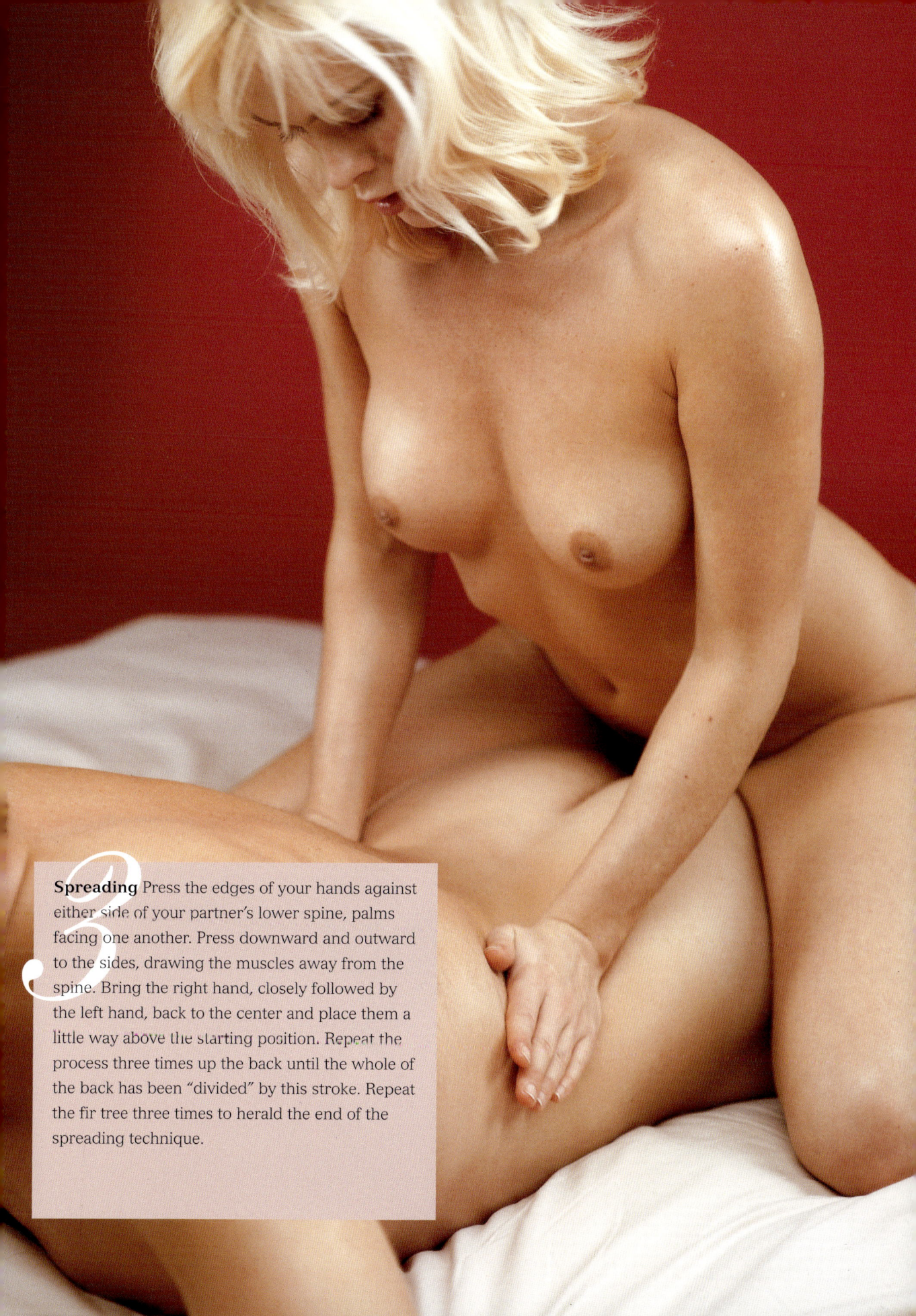

Spreading Press the edges of your hands against either side of your partner's lower spine, palms facing one another. Press downward and outward to the sides, drawing the muscles away from the spine. Bring the right hand, closely followed by the left hand, back to the center and place them a little way above the starting position. Repeat the process three times up the back until the whole of the back has been "divided" by this stroke. Repeat the fir tree three times to herald the end of the spreading technique.

Getting deeper

Now that you've warmed up your partner, you can start to build up the pressure and work more deeply on large muscle areas. The kneading techniques can produce deep waves of relaxation and stress relief if performed slowly and rhythmically, and will stimulate and invigorate if performed quickly. As you work, make sure your hands echo each other in a melody of alternating rhythms. Position yourself by your partner's right side for this part of the massage.

Pulling Place your left hand on your partner's left side at waist level, with your fingertips touching the floor or bed. Position your right hand slightly closer to your body. Now pull upward with the left hand and, just before it loses contact with the side of your partner's body, bring your right hand to the starting position to follow the trail of the left hand. Continue working in this way – using alternating hands to perform the stroke without ever losing contact with your partner's body – and work up along the side of the body. Repeat three more times, then do the same on the other side of your partner's body. Then repeat the entire sequence three more times.

Light kneading Kneading can be used to great effect on the soft muscles of the legs, buttocks, back, back of the neck, upper chest and upper arms. Reposition yourself at your partner's right side. Beginning on the left buttock and working up the left side of the body, grasp the flesh with one hand, squeeze without pinching and push it toward the other hand. Release the first hand then pick up and squeeze the flesh with the second hand. The action resembles kneading dough. It should be a smooth and flowing action that progresses up the back to the base of the neck, over the shoulders and out across the upper arms. Change position to work on the other side of the body.

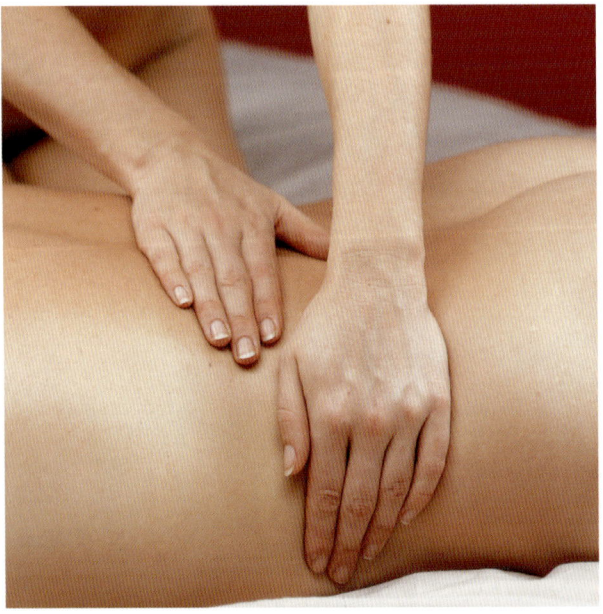
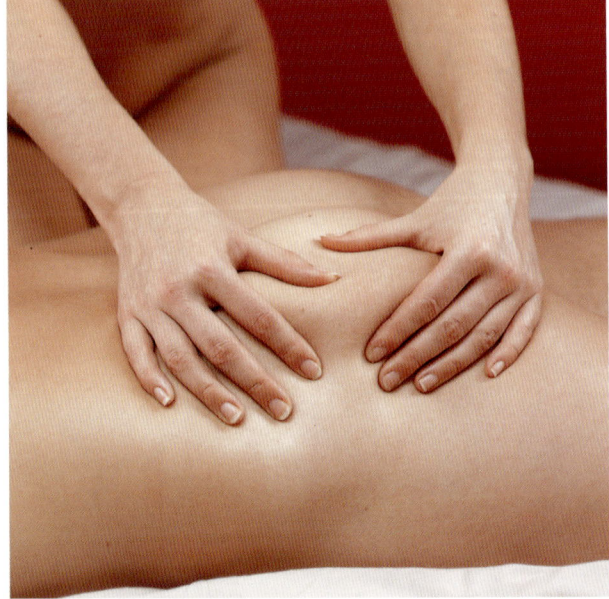

64 Stimulating & arousing

Deep kneading Return to your partner's right side. Place your palms side-by-side on the flesh on the left hip. Squeeze the flesh between both sets of index fingers and thumbs. There is often a handful to get hold of... Push the fingers away from each other, allowing the flesh to ease through the fingertips slightly, while making a zig-zag motion back and forth. Work thoroughly over the whole hip area, changing position if necessary to work on the opposite side of the body. Your kneading can be very deep and stimulating.

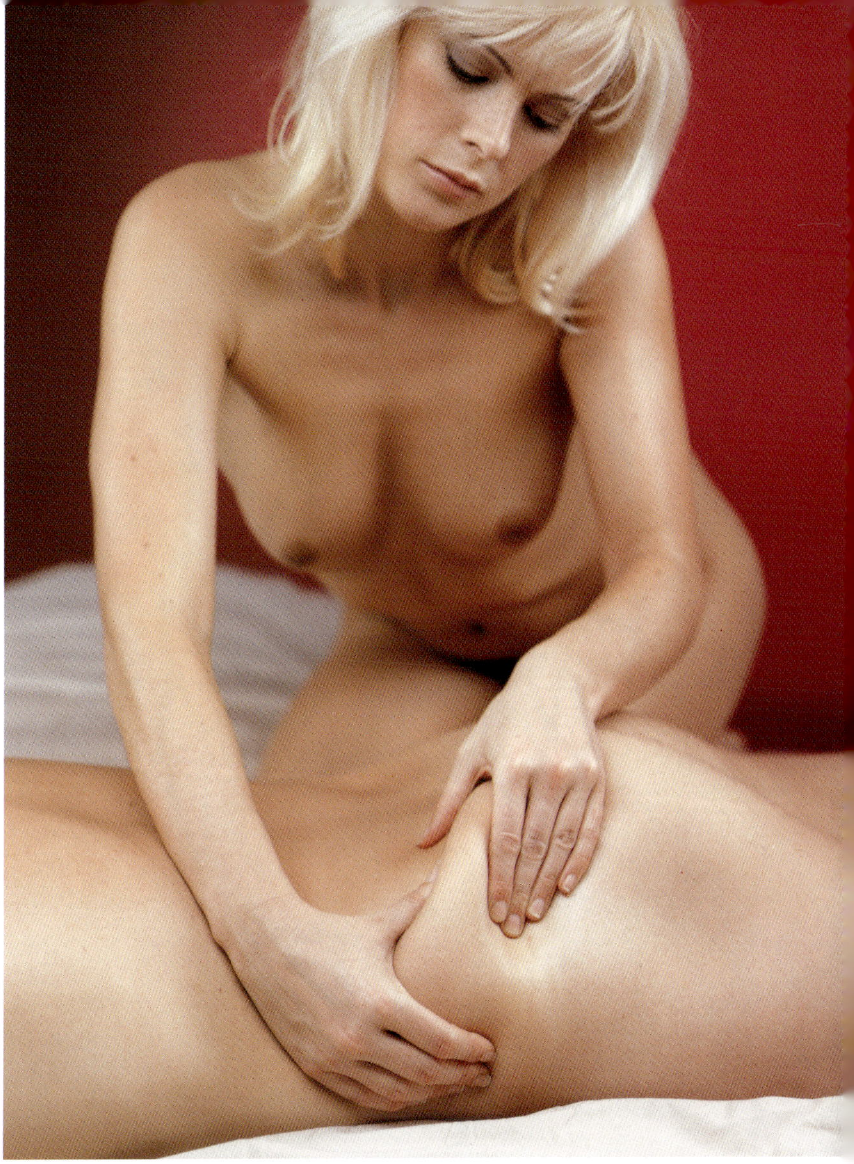

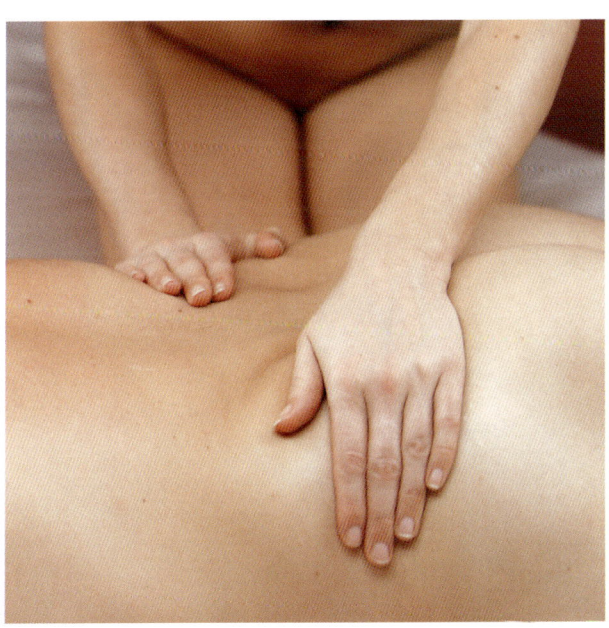

Crisscrossing Positioned back on your partner's right side, place your palms side-by-side on the flesh on the right hip. Push your right palm away from you in a horizontal strip across the back. As you pull your right hand back toward you, push your left hand away – they will pass by one another halfway, criss-crossing the body. Keep the hands moving constantly without leaving the surface of the skin, generating a warming friction as you perform this gathering/pushing technique. Allow the forearms to come into play as they make contact with the back and sides. Work your way up to the shoulders and back down to the hip, repeating as many times as you feel your partner needs it. Crisscrossing can also be performed gently over the front of the body from the pelvis to under the breasts.

Getting deeper

The spine

The massage so far has focused on the outside edges of the body, so now it is time to turn your attention to the center of the back – the muscles around the spine. This area holds a lot of tension. For these steps, straddle your partner's upper thighs, with the buttocks between your thighs.

1 Piano walking Imagine you are playing the piano on the shoulders and the soft muscle areas of the back. The pressure you apply depends on your personal strength, the comfort and pleasure feedback you get from your partner, and your intuition in the moment. Apply pressure from the tips of the fingers. Smooth off with interlaced fingers as shown in the Infinity Ribbon stroke (see pages 44–45). Do not use this technique if your fingernails are long enough to mark the skin.

Hot tip
The piano-walking technique is ideal for warming up your hands and your partner's body at the beginning of a massage sequence. After all, there's nothing more off-putting than cold hands!

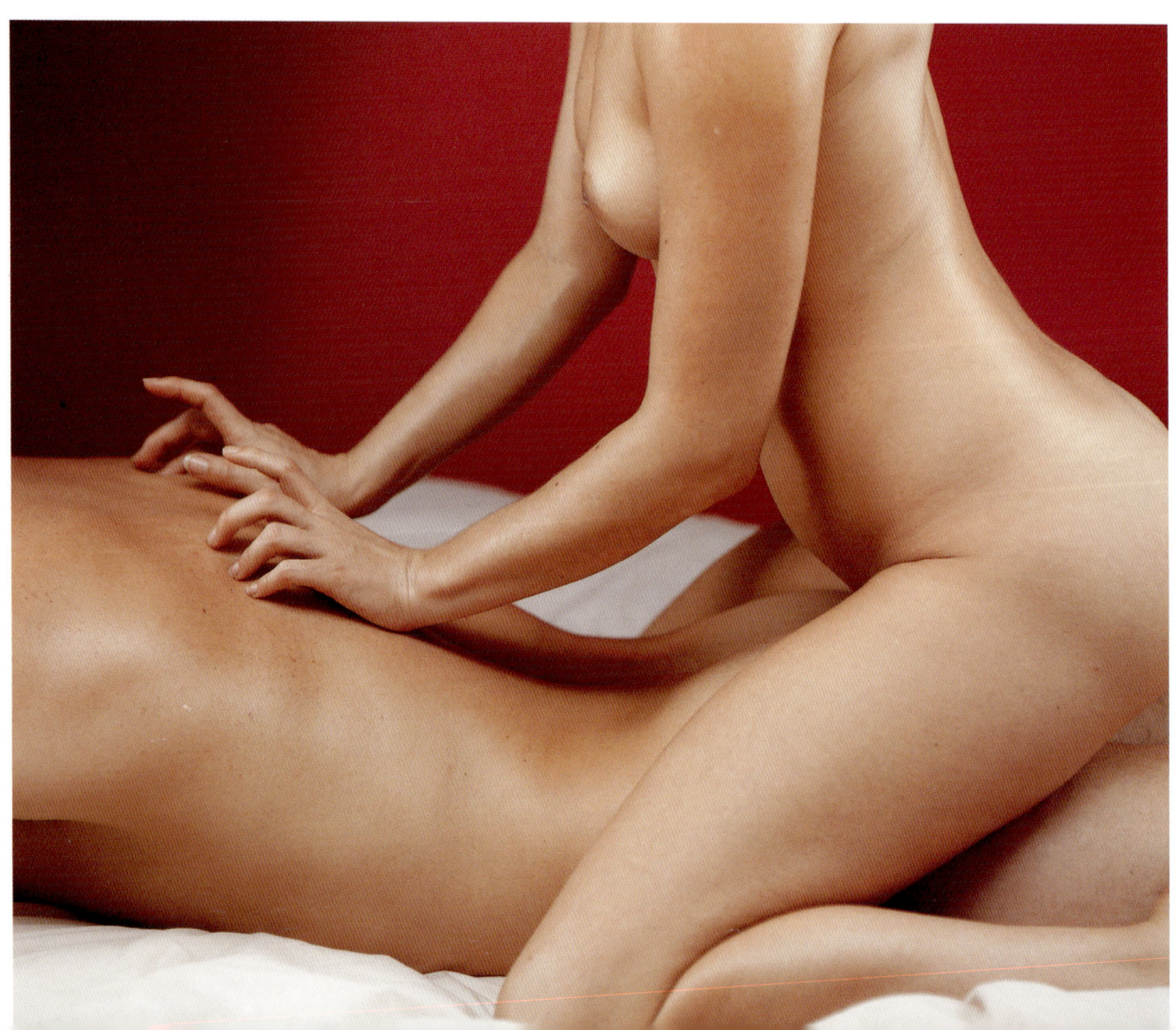

Edging Place the edges of the hands on either side of the top of the spine, resting the forearms along the back. Move your arms up and down a little way on either side of the spine (not directly on the vertebrae), slowly working your way from the neck to the tailbone. Repeat two or three times. If you wish, and if feedback from your partner is positive, continue edging over the buttocks and down the thighs. When working away from the spine, allow the palms to make contact with each other to increase the heat and friction. As well as generating a pleasing warmth in the muscles, the sound generated by the friction can have a soothing effect on the mind and emotions. Don't forget to use extra oil or talc to prevent chafing. Smooth off with gliding strokes.

Back-hand stroking This is a subtle stroke that can be overlooked in massage. The back of the hand represents the feminine touch while the palm represents the male touch. It is important, therefore, to use both sides of the hands in a massage sequence to create balance. Starting at the base of the back, position the backs of your hands on either side of the tailbone. Now simply trail the backs of the hands up along the body on either side of the spine, working toward the heart and, when you reach the top of the back, flip your hands over and pull your hands down the back resting on the palms. The forearms can also be incorporated into the stroke. Perform two or three times or as an interlude as you remember or mentally rehearse your next technique.

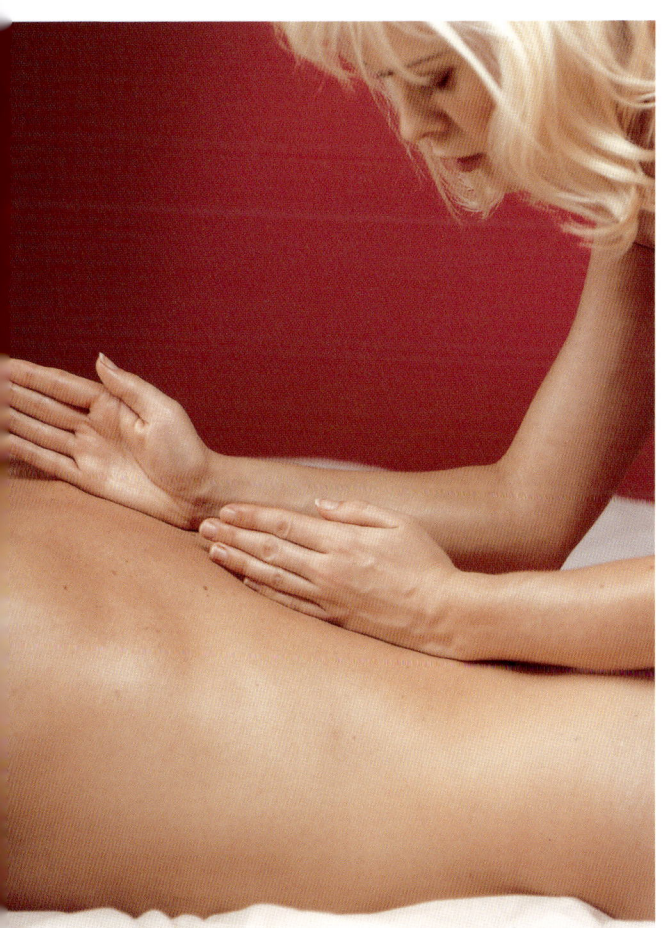
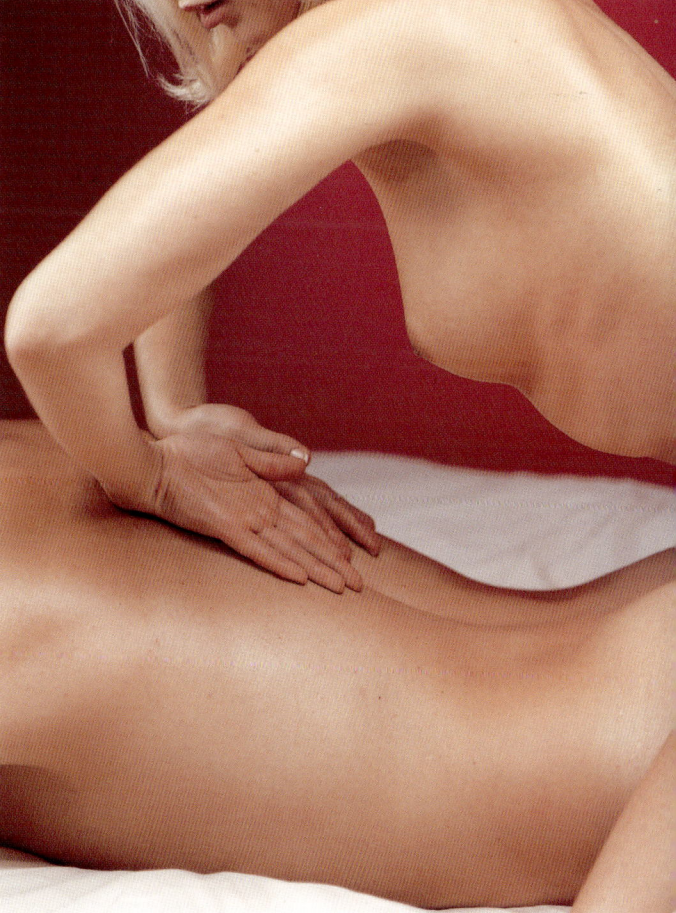

Varying the sensations

Stay in position, straddling your partner's thighs, for this part of the massage. The techniques shown here create a new range of sensations. They relax and relieve tension and can be highly arousing at the same time.

1 Raking Spread your fingers like flattened claws. Starting at the upper arms, work your way down both sides of the body (including buttocks and thighs, if you choose) using a raking motion, hand over hand. Vary the pressure to suit the texture of the skin and the thickness of the muscle. If your partner is very stressed this technique might induce a complete muscle group "shudder" and tension release, as the quick raking motion teases the large muscles to relax. Finish by smoothing off with gliding strokes.

Hot tip
Use a dry bristle bath brush or stiff hairbrush as an alternative to raking nails (especially if you don't have any!). Turn the brush over and smack the muscle areas to give a contrasting and stimulating sensation that might well be enjoyed!

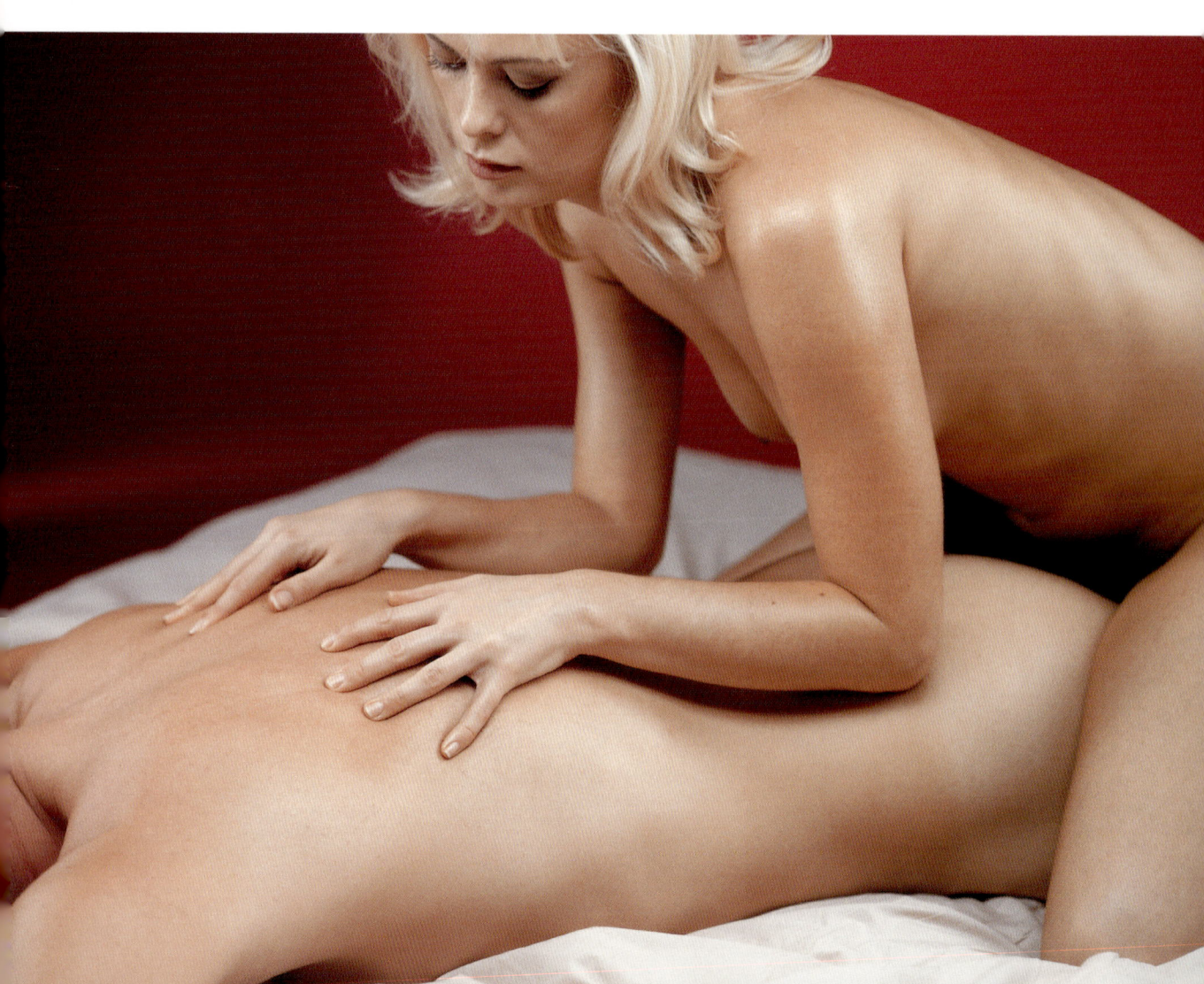

Scratching Men particularly appreciate this technique so, depending on the length and strength of your nails and the appetite of your partner, scratching can be done as strongly or as lightly as your recipient directs. As with raking, scratching brings blood to the surface, stimulating the circulation. It also has an arousing effect. Avoid this step if you have long or ragged nails.

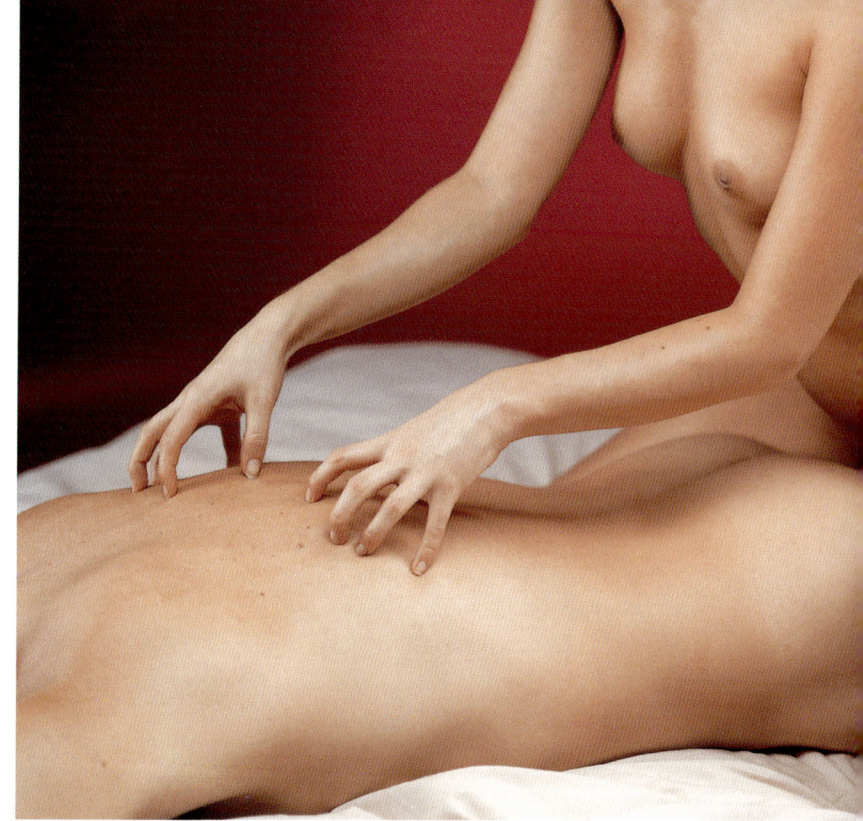

Rolling Starting at the lumbar region of the spine, grip the fleshy fold of skin on either side of the spine between the thumb and index finger of each hand (with either the thumb on top or vice versa, depending on the dexterity of your fingers). Roll the fold of flesh through your fingers, grasping it with first the fingers of the left hand, then with those of the right hand in turn, working your way up the back as far as possible. Some backs will be more pliable than others or offer you a greater or lesser amount of flesh to hold. Again, this technique will greatly stimulate blood flow and contribute to de-stressing and softening large muscle groups.

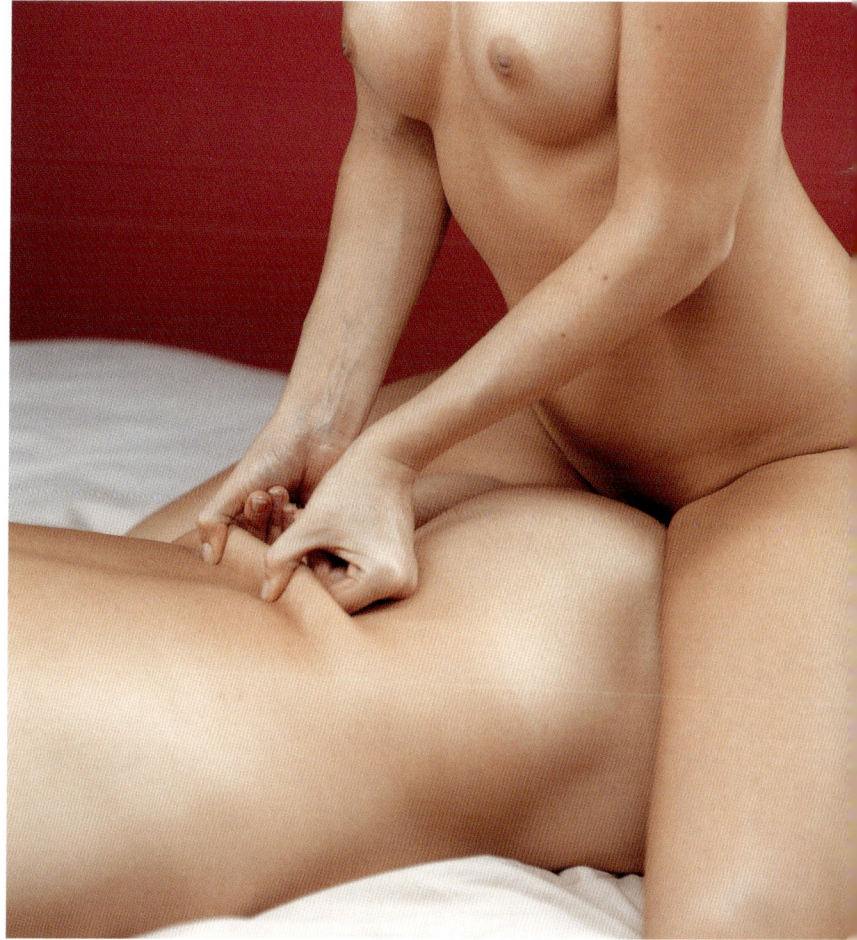

Working the buttocks

In our largely sedentary culture, a great deal of tension becomes stored in the large buttock muscles. Massage can often release long-held tension and bring relief. Laughter is often a consequence! Kneel astride your partner's knees for this part of the massage.

1 Squeezing Locate the hollows in the sides of the buttock muscles, situated slightly above and behind the point where the hip joint juts out. With fingers turned inward on the buttocks, lean forward while pressing into these hollows with the heels of the hands. Hold for a minute, then release. Repeat three times.

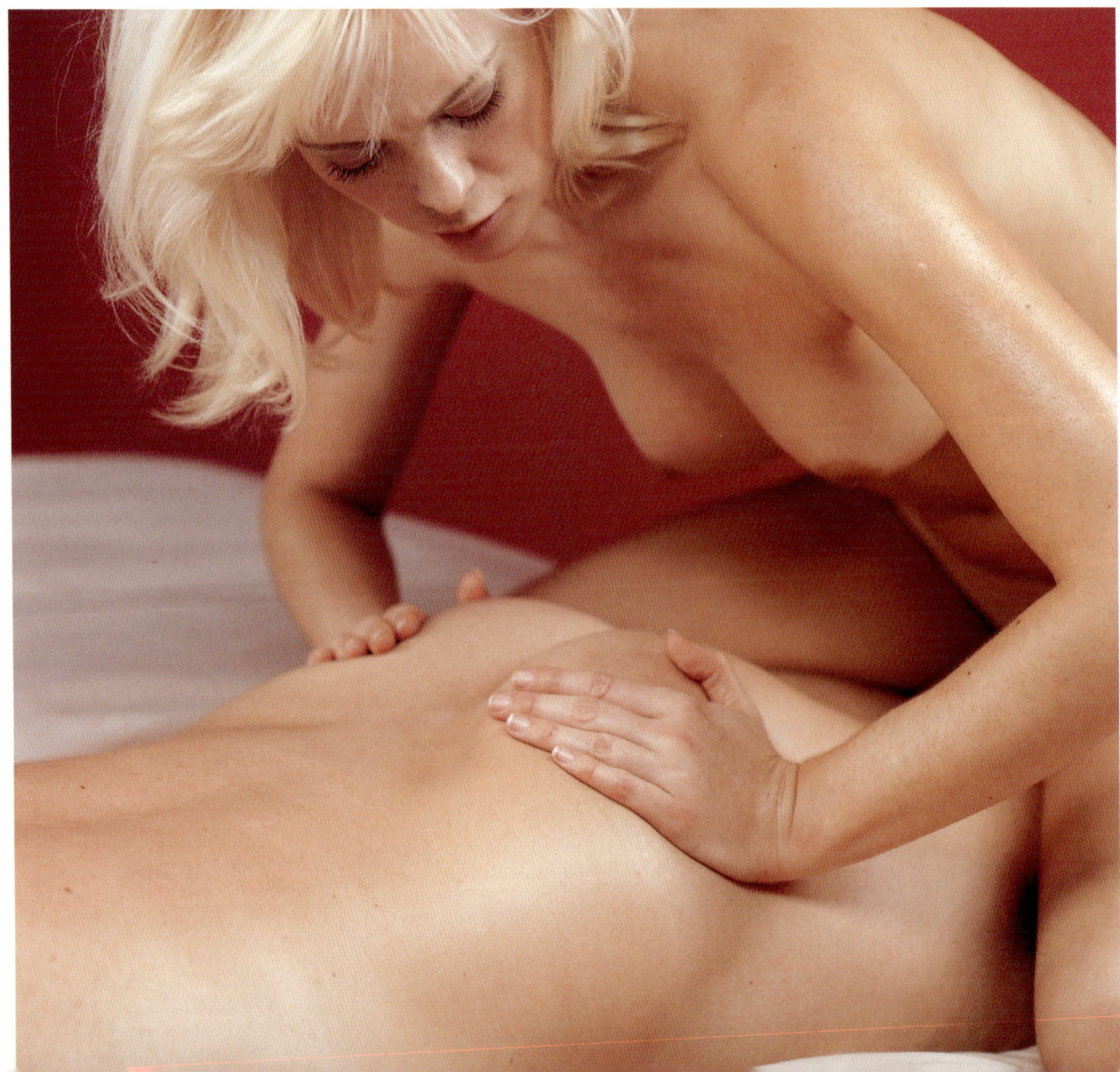

Elbow press Position your left elbow into the large buttock muscle on your partner's left buttock and lean your upper body into your arm to provide a strong downward pressure. Hold for two to three breaths, then ease your elbow down the side of the buttock about an inch and hold for another two to three breaths. Continue in this way until you reach the outer edge of the buttock, then repeat the whole process two to three times before finishing off with smooth strokes. Repeat with your right elbow on your partner's right buttock. If you wish to exert a lighter pressure, use your forearms instead of your elbows. With this technique you may like to work down the muscles in points along a vertical strip, close to the buttock crevice, down the middle of the muscle, then the outer edge. Move on to using both elbows at the same time by resting your chin in your hands to apply additional pressure.

Back press Start this technique at the very base of the spine near the crease in the buttocks on the pelvic girdle and finish between the shoulder blades. Place the heels of your palms on the muscles on either side of the spine. Now straighten your arms, inhale and, as you slowly exhale, lean your body weight into your hands. Inhale as you release the pressure, replace the hands a little higher up the back and, again, exhale slowly as you lean into your hands to press into the back. Allow the natural rise and fall of breath in your partner's rib cage to dictate your procedure to help create an empathetic union. Work up the back, then down again, and smooth off with gliding strokes. Repeat this step if you wish. Do not be disturbed if you hear small cracks and pops caused by vertebral realignment. Providing your partner does not suffer from back problems, this technique should provide welcome relief from muscular strain.

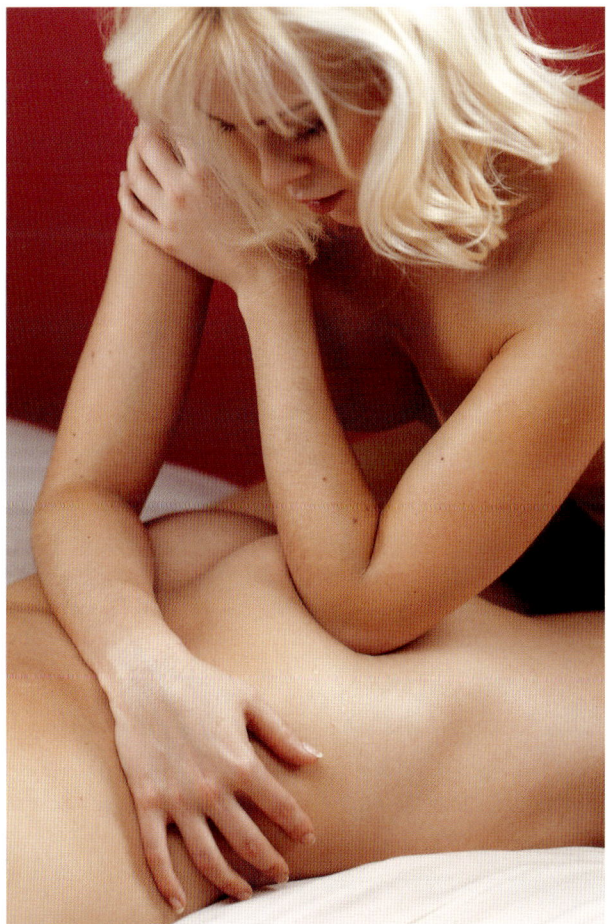
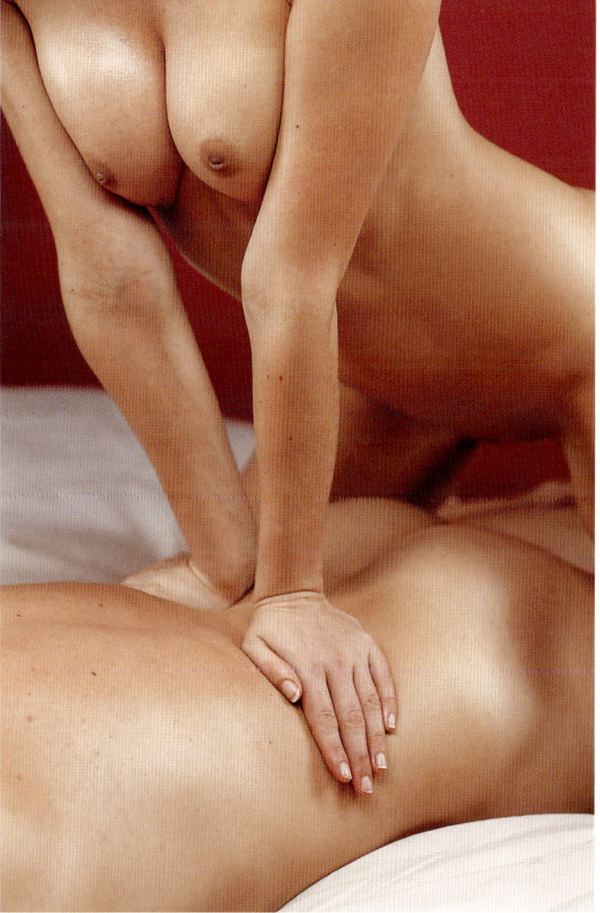

Working the buttocks

Smaller movements

You've made many sweeping and squeezing movements with the whole of the hand so far in this massage, so now it is time to use your thumbs and your knuckles for smaller, more focused movements. You should still be sitting astride your partner, now at the top of the thighs.

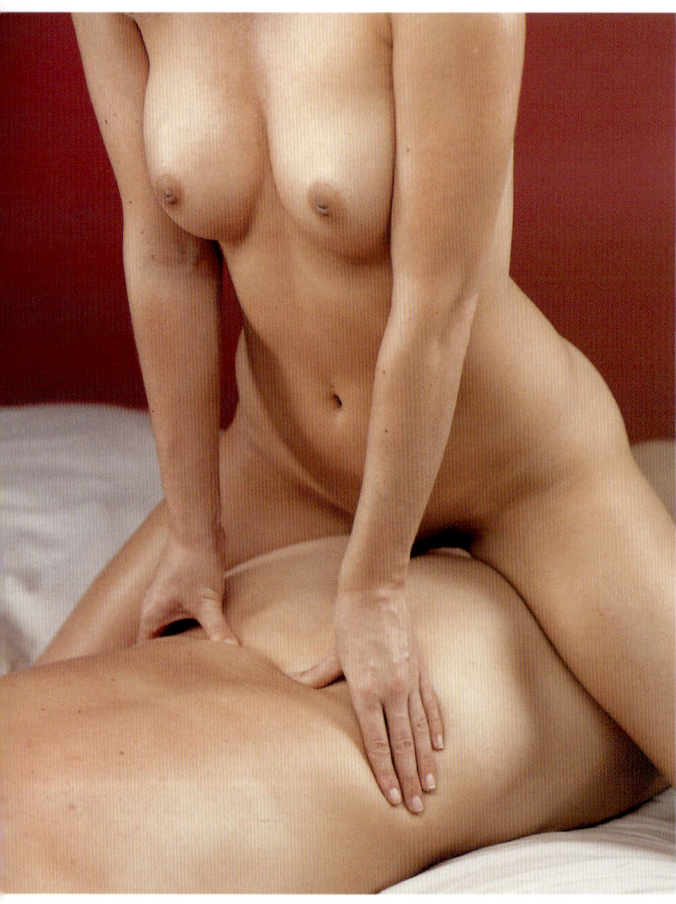

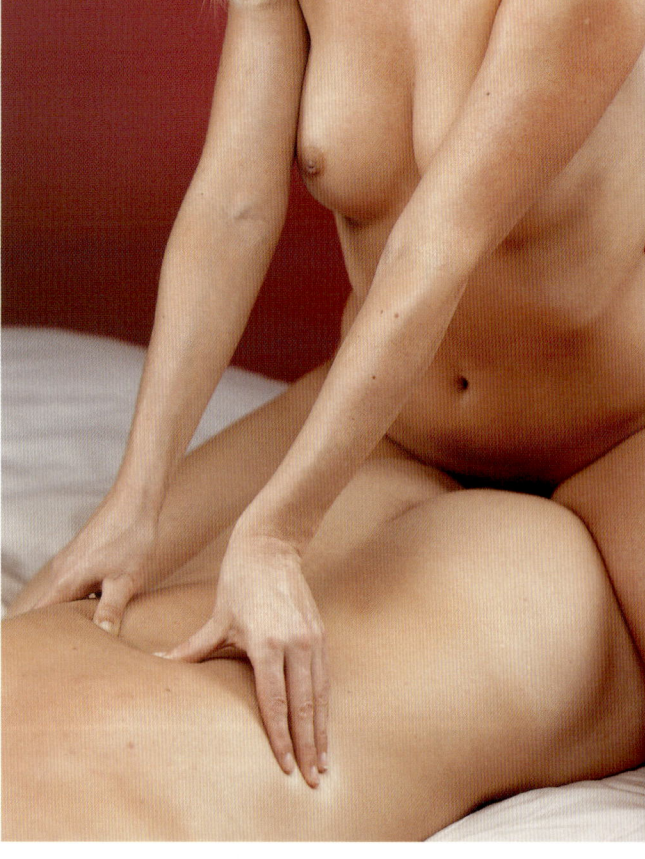

Thumb press Place your thumbs on the pads of muscle to either side of the lower spine, just above the pelvis. Attune yourself to your partner's breathing and lean your body weight into your thumbs during an exhalation (exhaling yourself at the same time). Hold momentarily then inhale as you release the pressure and move the thumbs a thumb's width up the back. Continue as far as you can manage comfortably from your starting position, but note that the technique should not extend into the neck region.

Circular thumb pressure Similar to the thumb press, and starting and finishing in the same areas, substitute simple downward pressure for a robust outer circling of the thumbs. As ever, adjust your touch and pressure to the preferences of your partner (light or firm), working your way up and down the back and smoothing off with plenty of gentle finishing strokes.

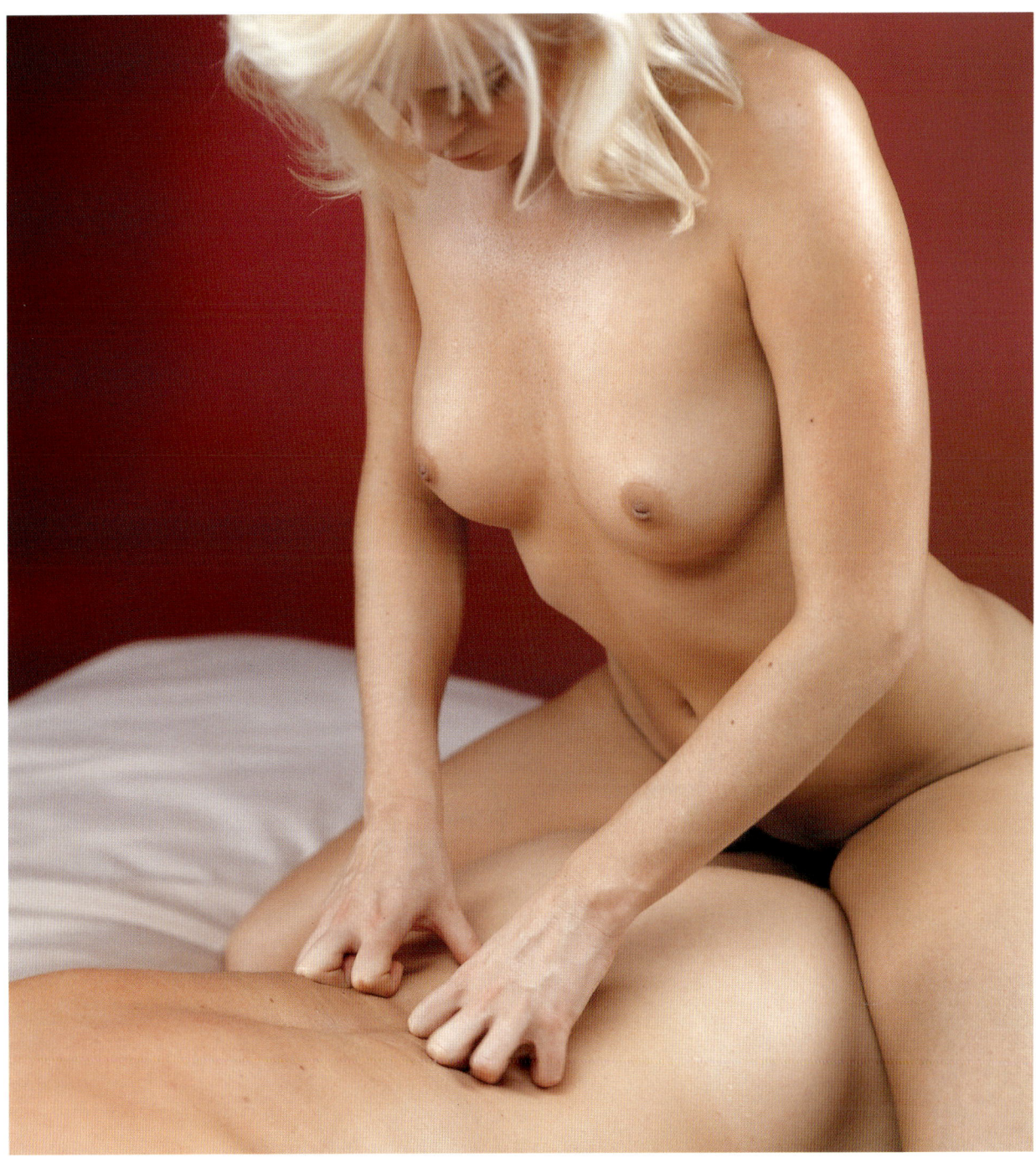

Knuckling Use the knuckles in a "gathering" motion to work on the muscles farther away from the spine. Your thumbs will anchor each position as you progress along the length of the back. Be aware of your partner's breath and look out for verbal or postural feedback. Follow this step by smoothing off with plenty of gentle finishing strokes.

Invigorating moves

The following techniques are robust and invigorating, and will help to stimulate and revitalize your partner. Be sure to attune yourself to your partner's responses and adjust the pressure that you use accordingly as you could easily apply too much pressure for his comfort with these vigorous techniques. Make sure that you don't hack or perform any percussion strokes behind the kneecap. Position yourself at your partner's right side at waist level.

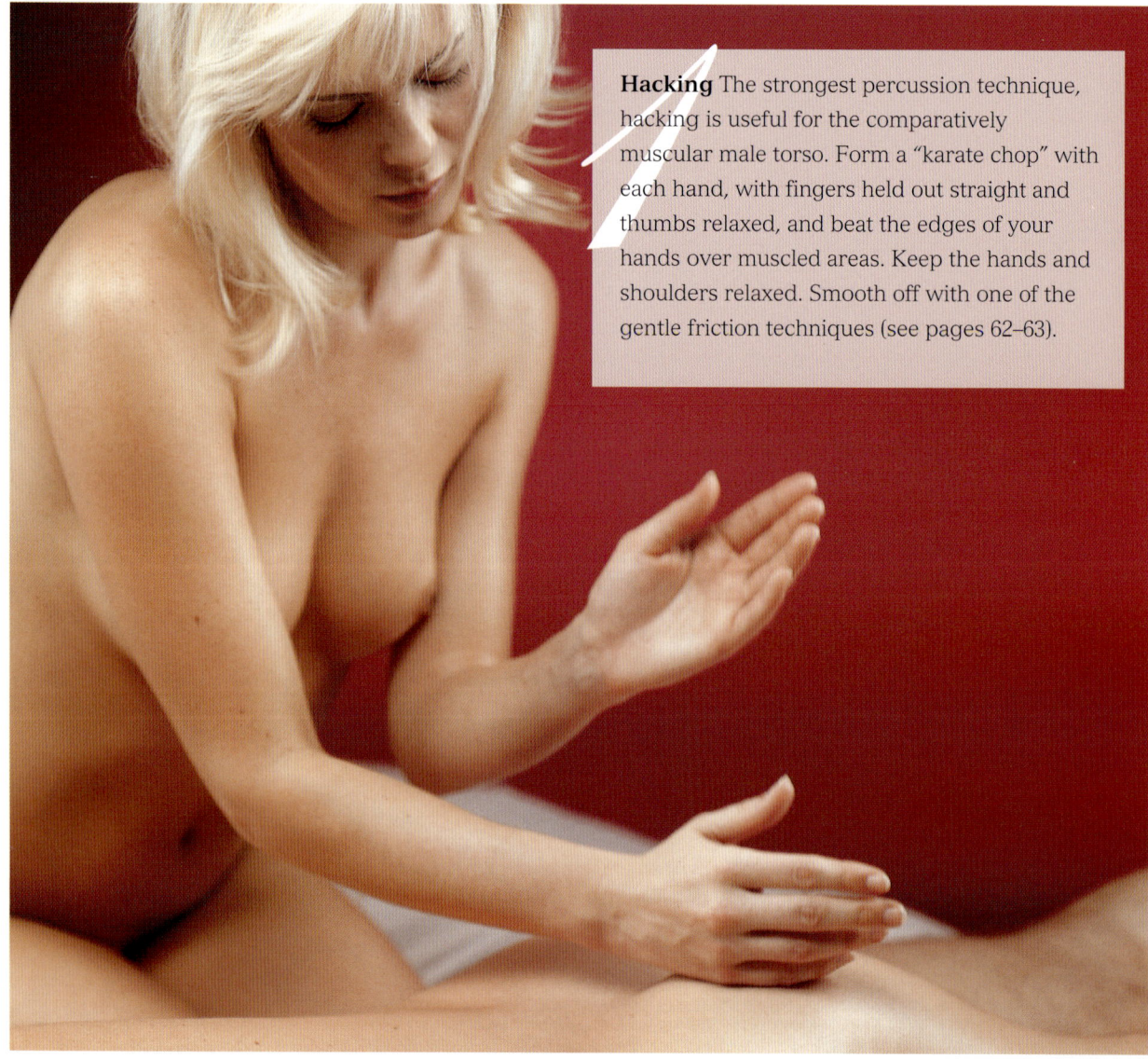

1 Hacking The strongest percussion technique, hacking is useful for the comparatively muscular male torso. Form a "karate chop" with each hand, with fingers held out straight and thumbs relaxed, and beat the edges of your hands over muscled areas. Keep the hands and shoulders relaxed. Smooth off with one of the gentle friction techniques (see pages 62–63).

Pummeling Starting at the heavily muscled buttocks, and with your hands forming fists, beat your hands against the skin alternately in a rhythmic fashion as you work up and down the back, arms and legs. Smooth off with a gentle finishing stroke.

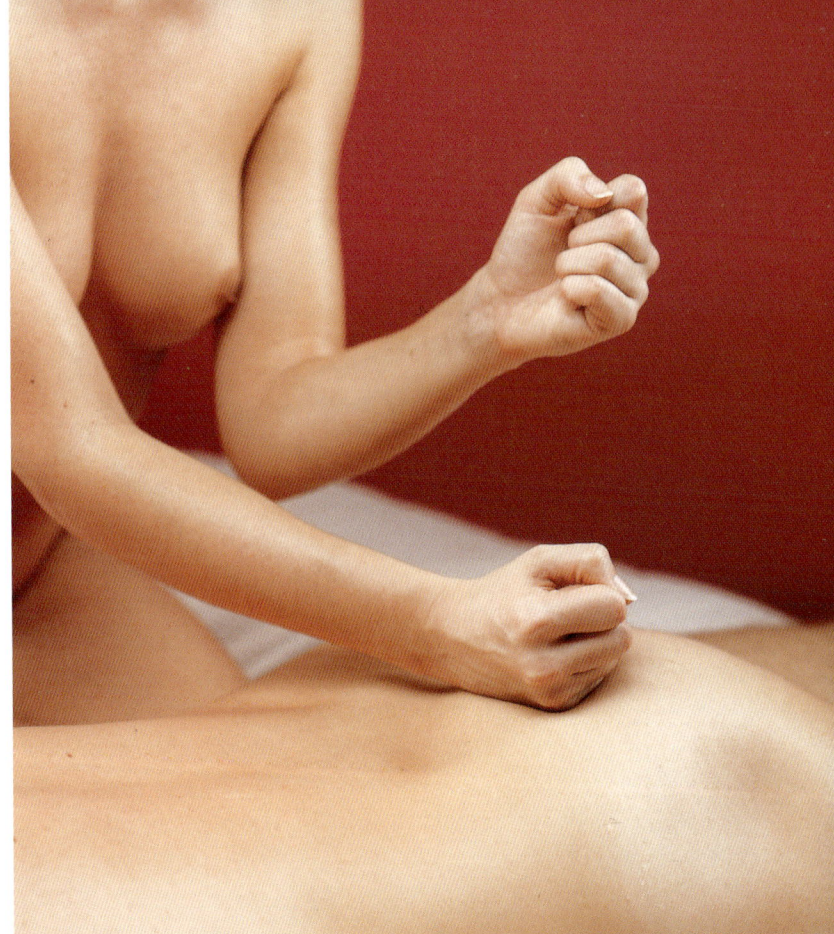

Cupping This is a rapid sequence of alternate drumming strokes formed by your cupped hands trapping air against the skin. Particularly when performed directly on the skin, rather than through clothing, it makes a loud "popping" sound when the hand leaves the skin and the trapped air escapes. Arch your hands at the knuckles, keeping your fingers straight, and "cup" the area you are working on, using the hands rapidly and alternately. Work methodically across the entire back, paying attention to your partner's comfort. Thirty seconds or so should suffice for most treatments. Smooth off with one of the gentle friction techniques. Although this technique may seem dramatic, it will not hurt at all if performed correctly.

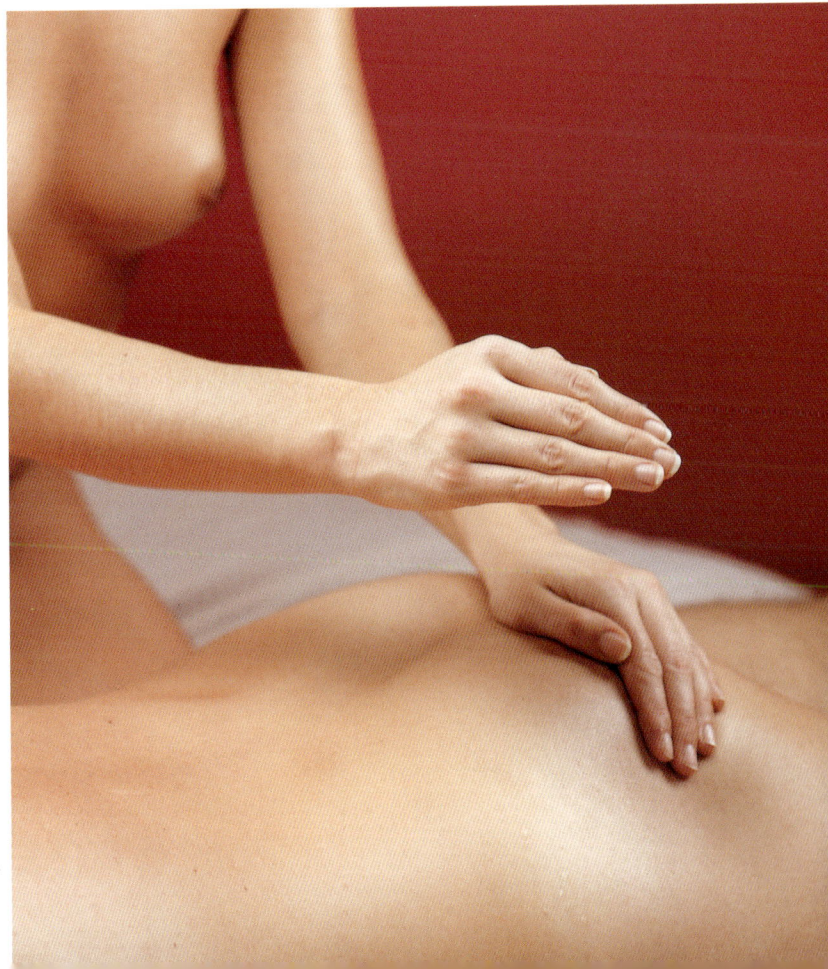

Enlivening the skin

Stay in position, at your partner's right side, for these stimulating techniques that focus on the nervous sensations just beneath the skin's surface. They can make the skin tingle and feel fresher and help to release nervous ticks and afflictions. For any readers familiar with Thai massage, the rhythmic one-two-three-pause sound of the clicking technique might well evoke happy memories of Thai beaches.

Plucking Grasping a segment of flesh between the thumb and index finger of each hand, work your way over areas of the back that have skin and flesh enough to spare. Like other stimulating techniques, this will invigorate passive muscles and revitalize the skin. Smooth off with gentle finishing strokes. For added pleasure, pluck with your fingertips on the looser, fuller, muscled areas. Hold for a second then release and repeat.

Clicking Lightly press your palms together, overlapping the thumbs and splaying the fingers slightly. Beat downward with the edges of the little fingers using a one-two-three-pause rhythm, allowing the fingers to "click" as they close together. Perform this technique over the chosen muscle area, then smooth off with a gently soothing stroke. With care, clicking can even be performed lightly over the head.

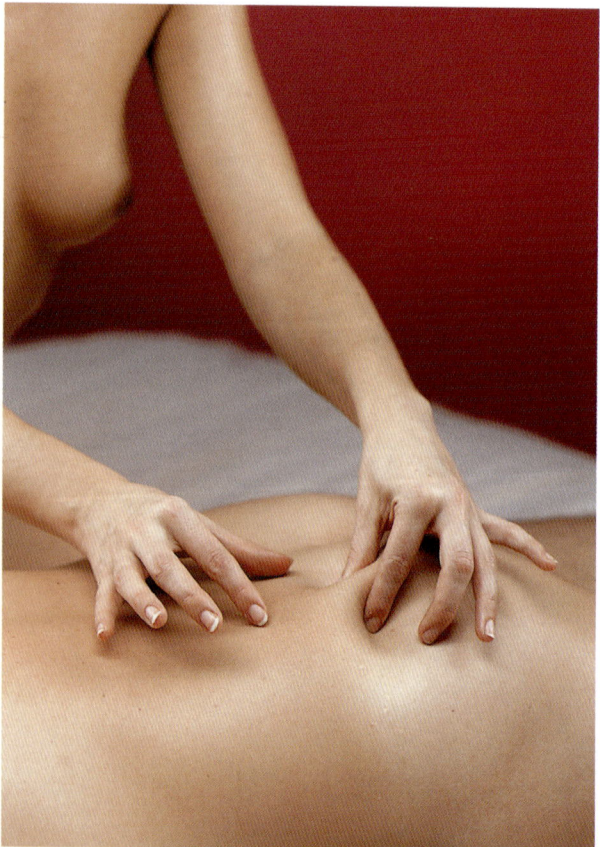
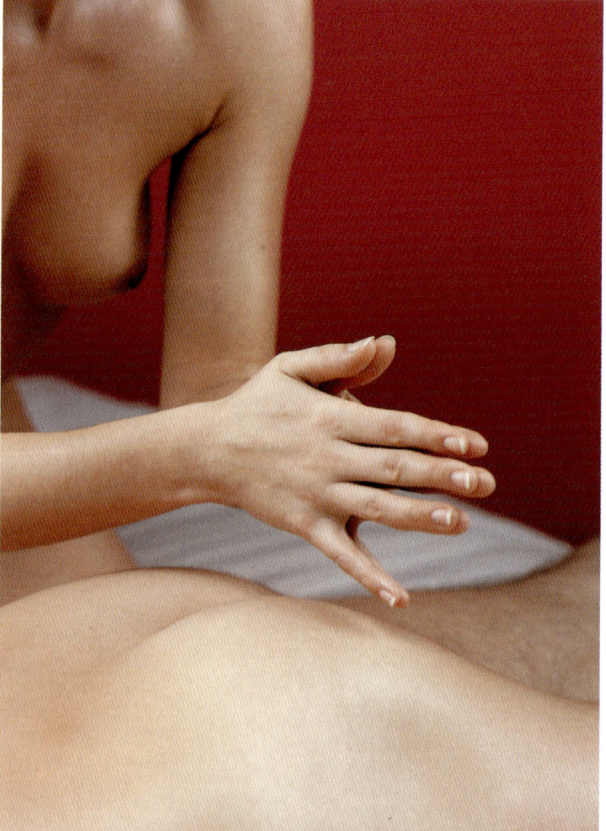

3 Smacking This technique is just as you would imagine, but with two variations. The first is a light stroke with the fingers slightly relaxed, made in a rapid succession over any muscled area, and can be rather pleasant once you establish your partner's tolerance level. Finish off with comforting, smoothing strokes. Smacking in this way dilates blood vessels and warms cold and sedentary muscles. The second variation is a well-established favorite of erotic game-play. Without warning, deliver a stinging, full-handed smack to either one or both buttocks. You'll have to judge when the moment might be just right and be prepared for a range of possible reactions from your partner. If it doesn't go down well, a loving, soothing massage apology should cover your actions. If it does … well, it might move you on in almost any direction!

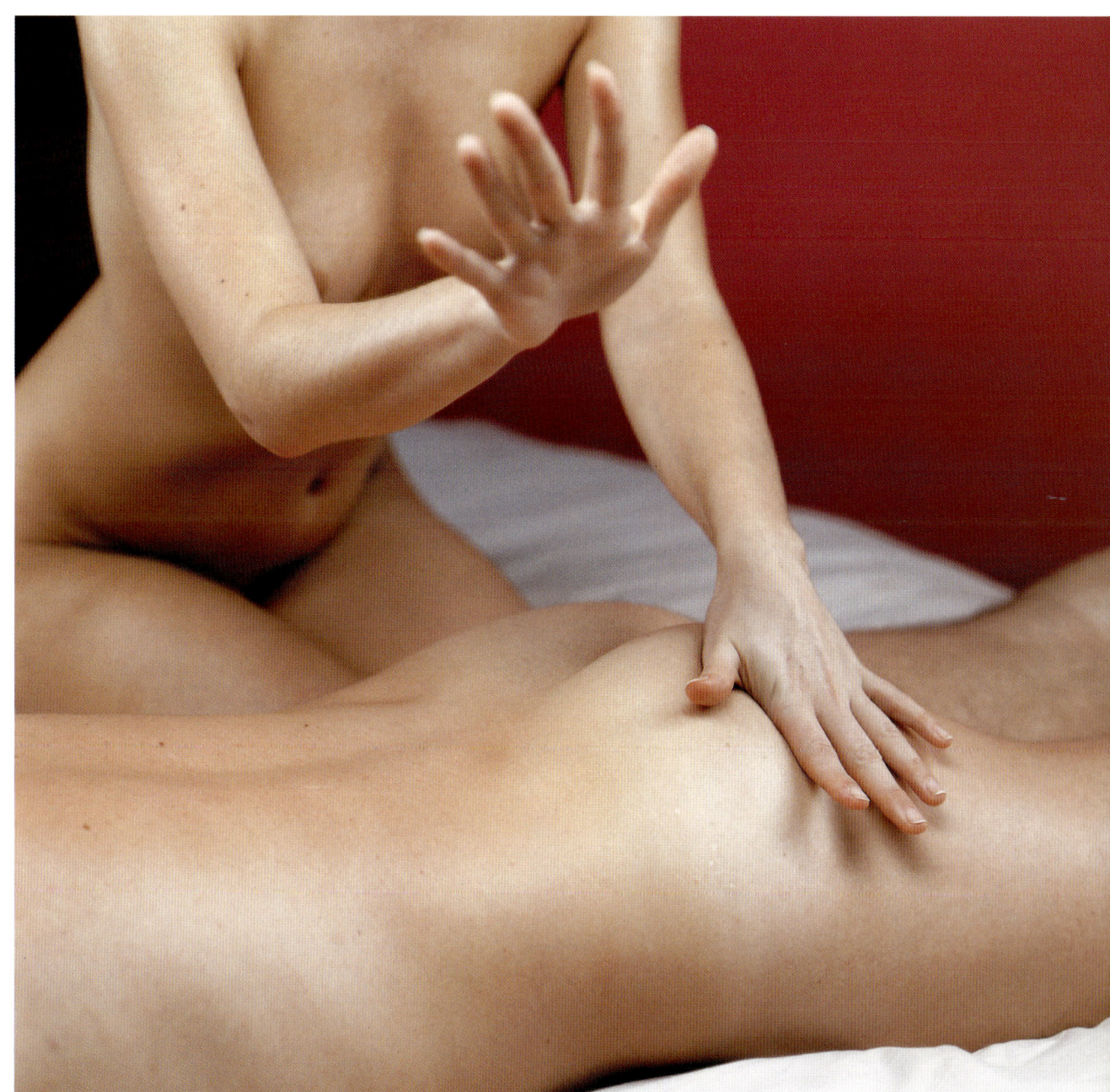

Enlivening the skin

Body moves

Up until now your hands have done all the work, but now it is time to put your entire body into the massage. The techniques here are dramatic to look at and are wonderful to receive as this massage draws to a close, although they should be avoided if your partner has any back problems, particularly a distorted spine.

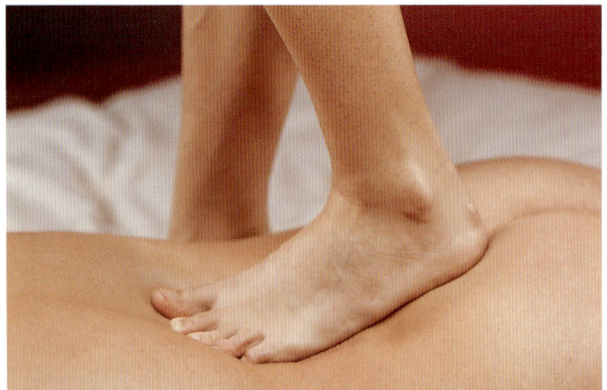

Foot rocking Stand astride your partner's legs with your feet rooted firmly on the ground, yet with a sense of lightness in all your body as it aspires toward the heavens. Place one foot on the lower spine between the buttocks and apply very light pressure. Gently rock your partner's body from side to side with your foot, soothing him into a state of relaxation. Repeat this motion five or six times or until you feel your partner has released tension or stiffness. Eventually you will sense when your partner has let go and handed the power of movement over to you.

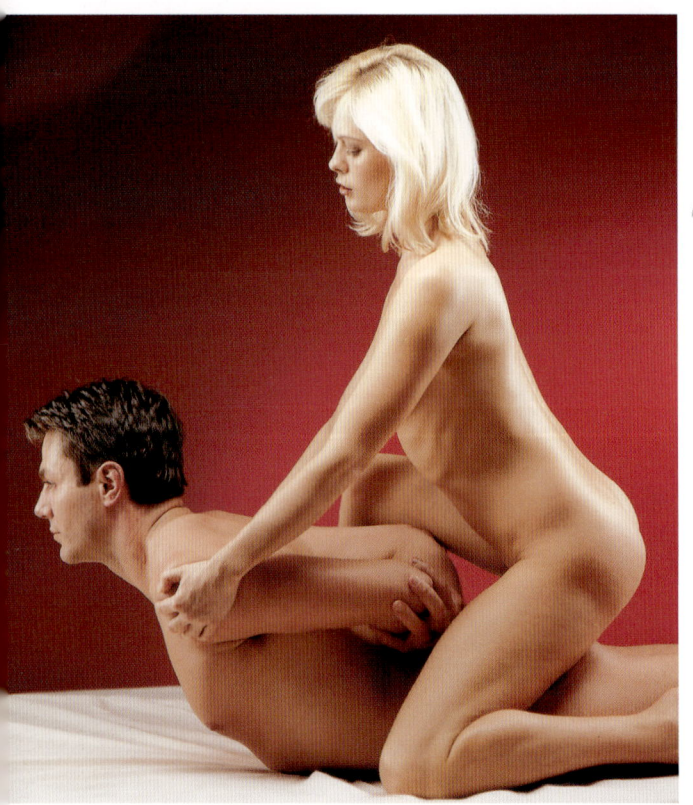

Chest expanding This technique provides all-round benefits and is excellent for people with poor posture, asthma, bronchitis, breathing problems or lack of body tone. Sit astride your partner's legs. Bend your right knee and place your right foot on the floor to brace your body during the movement to come. Ask your partner to grasp his forearms or elbows behind the back. With both hands, securely cup your partner's shoulder joints. Once again, synchronize your breathing with your partner's and, on an inhalation, slowly pull back the shoulders until the muscles offer resistance (try and learn to be sensitive to the limitations of the muscles so you don't pull back too far). Hold a position that will allow both of you to breathe comfortably for three to four complete breaths, then slowly relax and release the posture as your partner rolls down onto the floor. Take a few breaths before repeating two to three times. There is often a wonderful sense of revitalized energy flow associated with the release of this posture.

Stimulating & arousing

Hip swaying Make sure that your partner is relaxed before you perform this technique. Standing astride the upper legs, bend your knees and lean over your partner's body to cradle the hip bones firmly in your hands. Synchronize your breathing with your partner's and, on the next exhalation, lift the hips a little way off the ground. Your partner's knees should remain on the floor. Ensure you have the body's full dead weight in your hands. If your partner still seems a little stiff, shift the weight slightly to left and right to encourage him to let go. Hold for three to four complete breaths. Relax and release the position, supporting the hips as you lower them gently to the floor. You must be confident in both your position and your ability to hold your partner's weight comfortably, or he will not trust you enough to let go. Remember that incorrect lifting can damage your back. Make sure you keep your knees bent at all times and do not lock them. Use the power of the thigh muscles to do the actual lifting – there should be no strain involved.

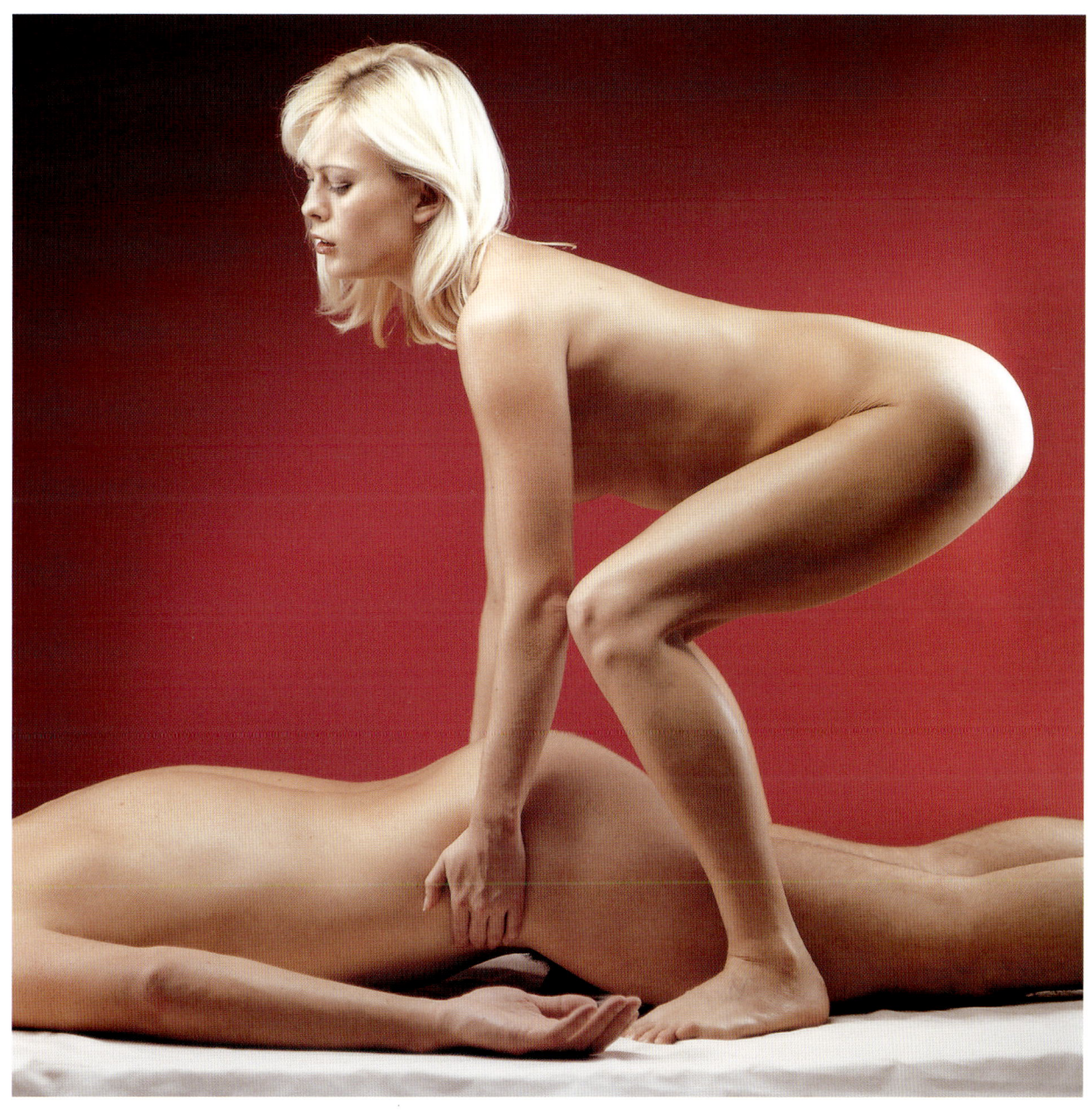

Stretches

By now your partner should be feeling both relaxed and energized. End the massage with these luxurious body stretches. Your partner's body will feel lighter, longer and more alive as you bring your stimulating and arousing massage to a close.

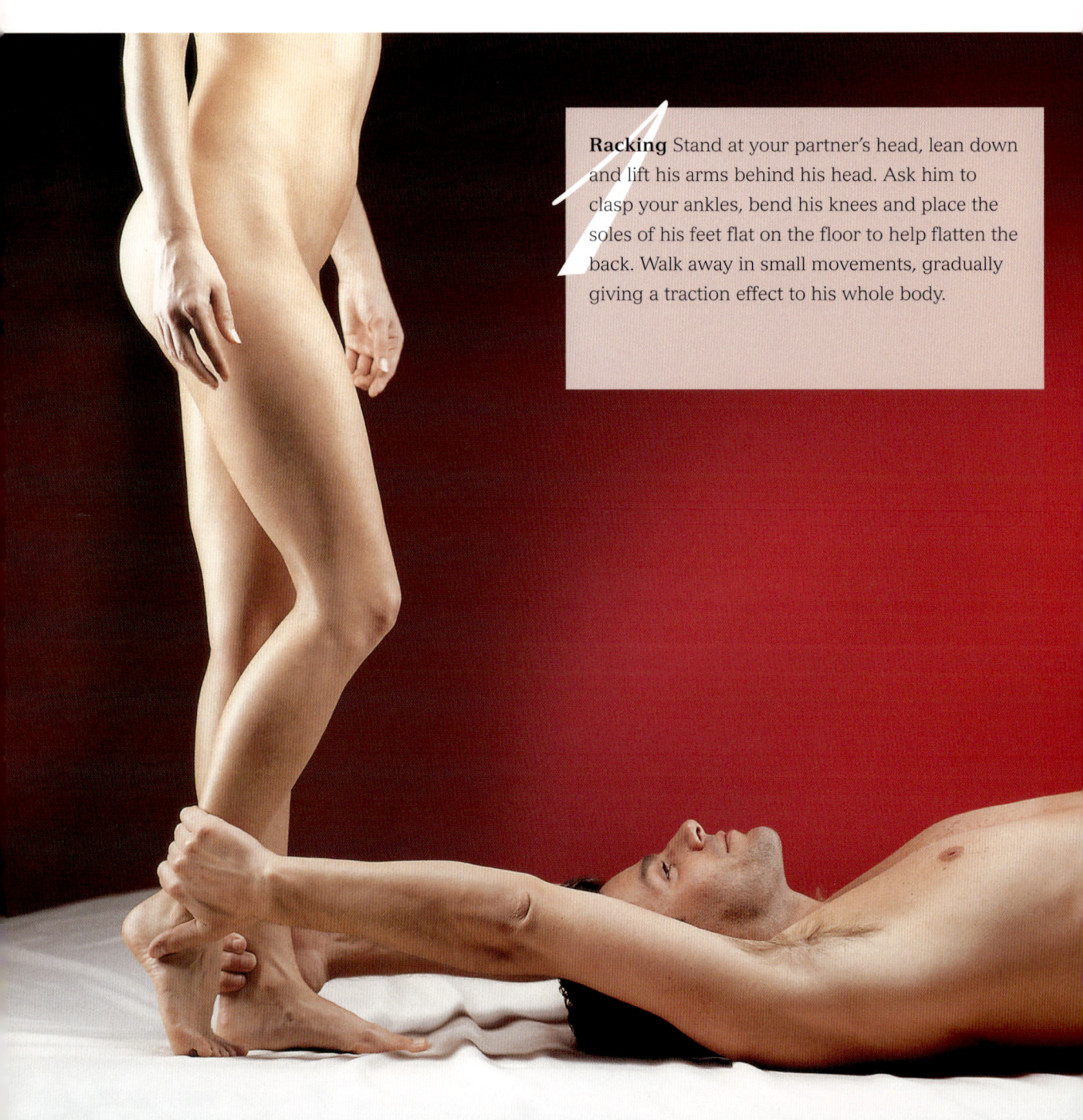

1 Racking Stand at your partner's head, lean down and lift his arms behind his head. Ask him to clasp your ankles, bend his knees and place the soles of his feet flat on the floor to help flatten the back. Walk away in small movements, gradually giving a traction effect to his whole body.

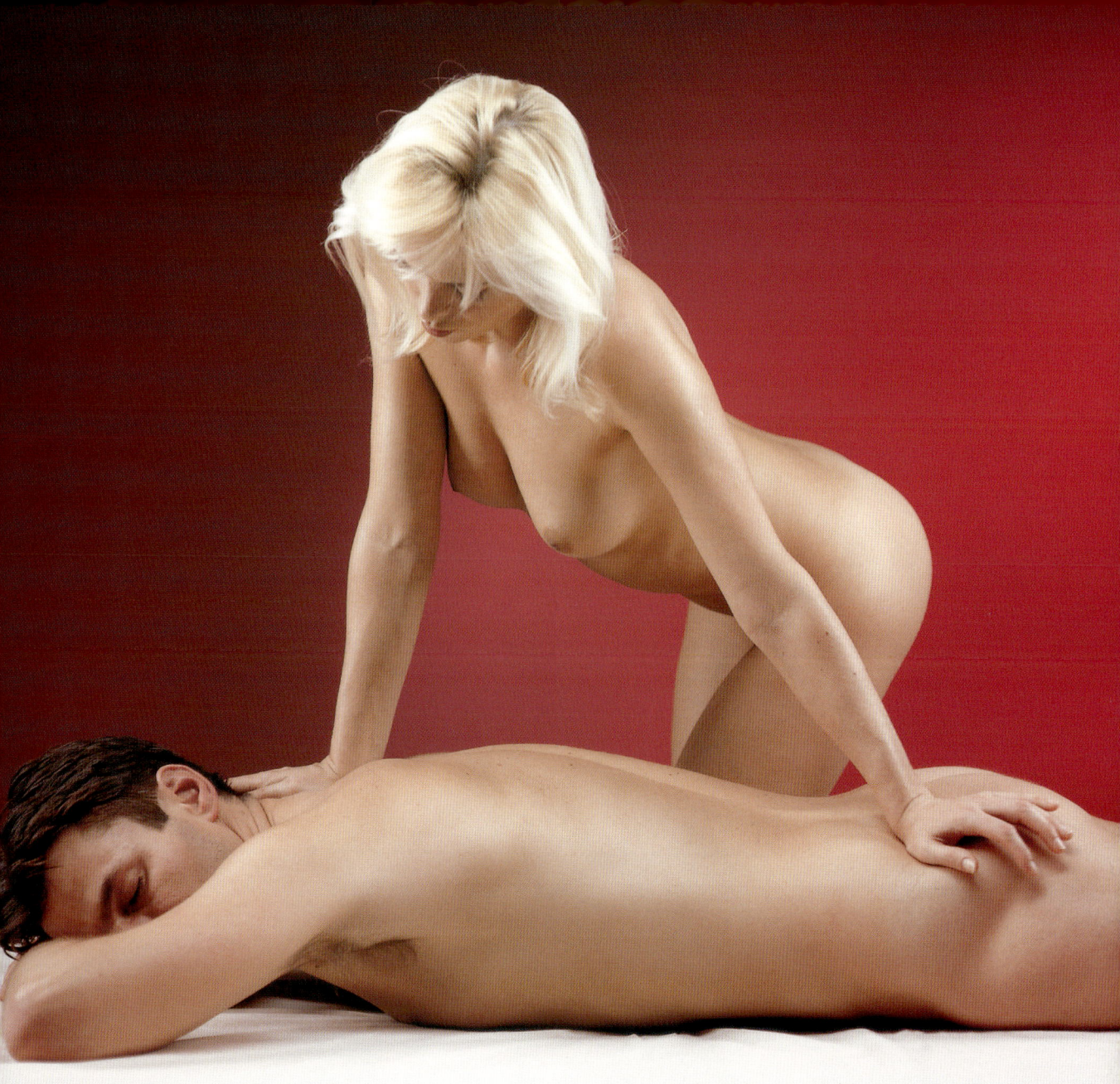

Cross-stretching Kneel down on your partner's right side at hip level and place your right (dominant) hand on the right shoulder blade and your left (supporting) hand on the top of the left buttock. (Reverse the sides if you are left-handed.) Inhale, then exhale as you push both hands away from each other in a diagonal stretch across the body. This may well force your partner to exhale, so when you sense that he needs to inhale, do so yourself as you release the pressure. Repeat two or three times then either work from the other side of the body or move your hands to the opposite shoulder and buttock. Repeat three or four times.

Hot tip

As a final, loving gesture, slowly cover your partner with a warmed sarong or blanket. Over this covering, with one or two hands, smooth around the whole body in a clockwise direction. To finish, rest one hand on the heart area or between the shoulder blades.

Stretches 81

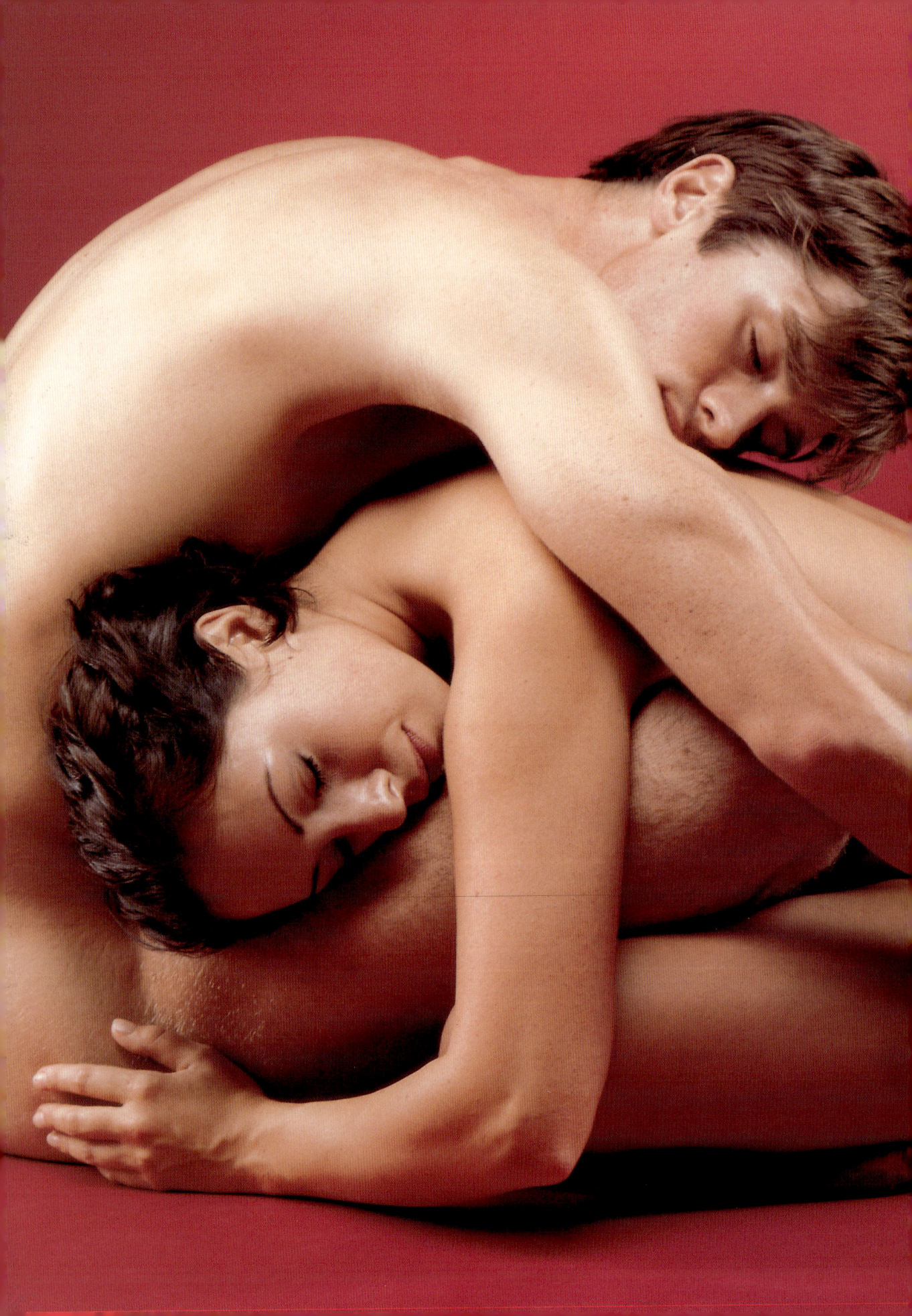

Beyond skin deep

Get ultra close and personal with this series of statuesque Thai postures – sculptured re-creations of classical erotic positions that work on deep-seated muscles and joints. Build up your stamina and prowess and make beautiful shapes together.

Thai bodywork

This chapter features a sequence of techniques from Thai bodywork. This physical workout requires an attunement of both body and breathing between you and your partner, where two become one – an almost mystical union where you are not sure where your skin ends and another's begins. It is an ideal way for two lovers to come together.

Back warmer If you've always wanted to walk over your partner, here's your chance! Seat your partner on a comfortable cushion that raises the hips slightly and helps to correct the spine and posture. He may cross his legs or have them resting in an "open diamond" shape. Sit behind your partner on a cushion, an arm's length away. Ask your partner to reach back with his arms. Clasp one another's wrists and place your feet on the muscles on either side of the base of your partner's spine. Walk your feet up the muscles on either side of the spine in small increments. At the same time, pull gently on the arms. Lighten the pressure at the upper part of the back, between the shoulder blades, by pressing with the toes and the pads (either heels, balls or toes, depending on your comfort) of the feet. This step provides a general warm-up for the back muscles and is great for relieving lumbago and lower back stiffness.

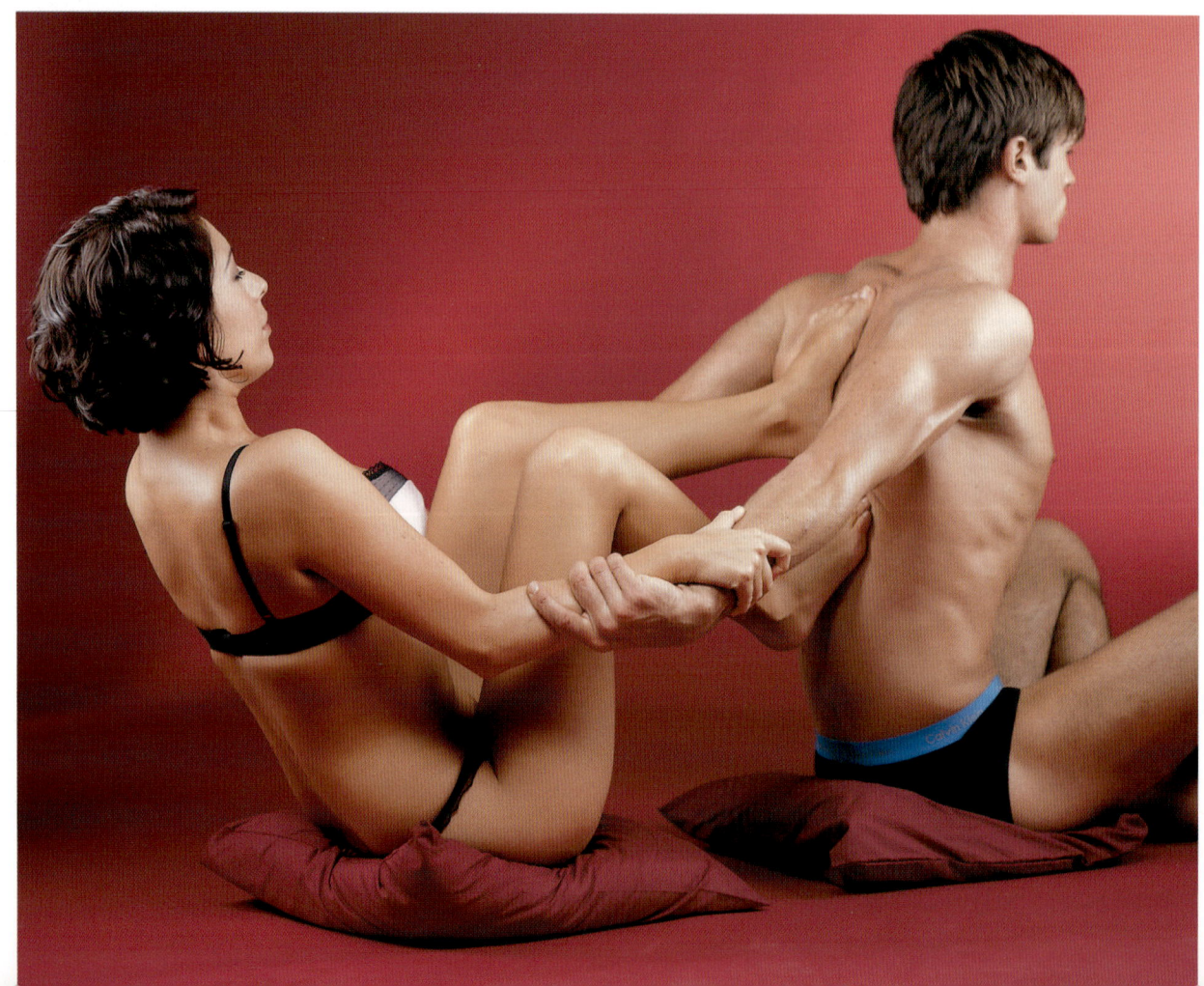

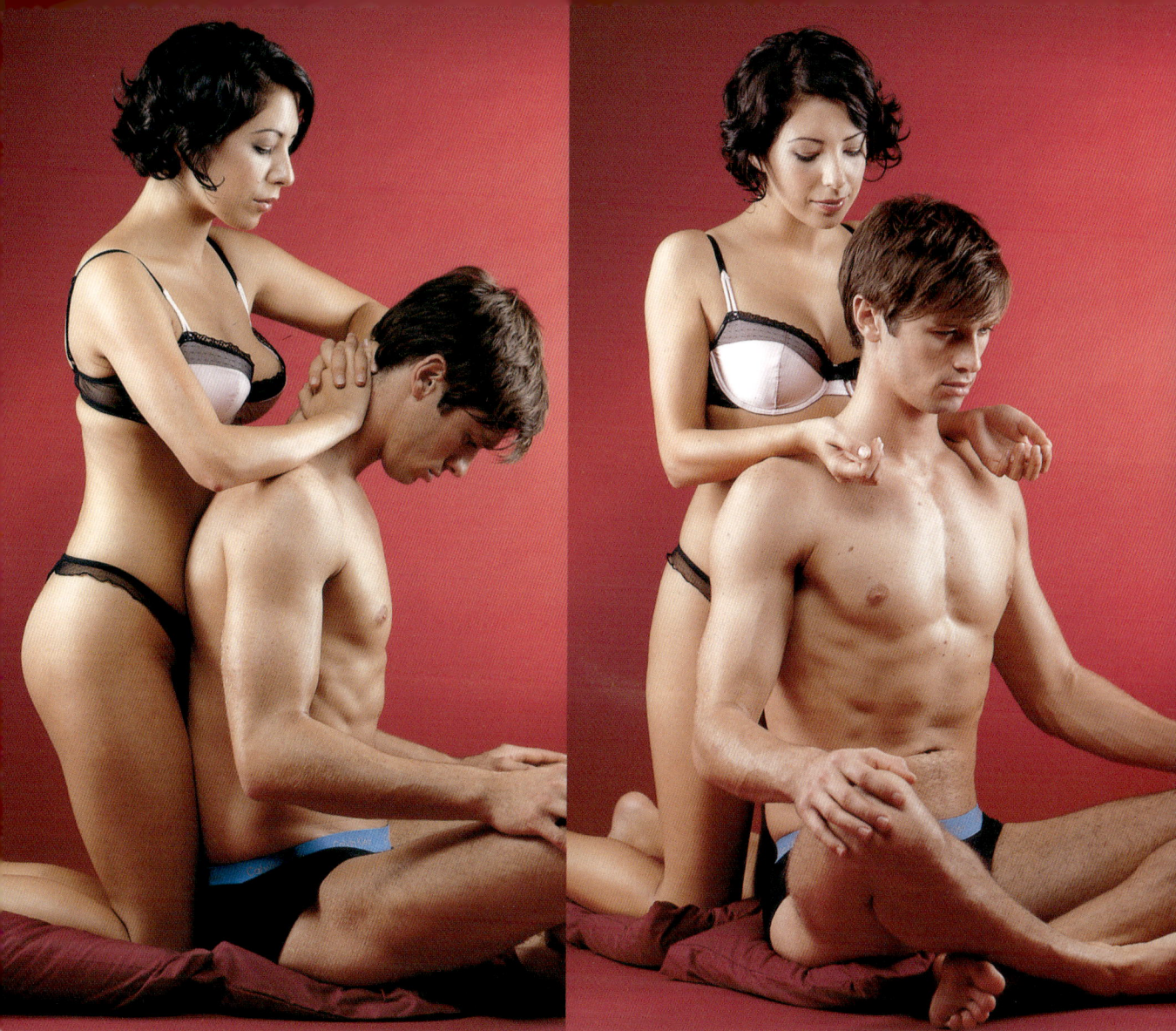

Neck and shoulder press Kneel behind your partner with your thighs close against his back and place the palms of your hands on the trapezius muscles at the top of his shoulders. Inhale, then exhale as you press down with the heels of the hands in three distinct positions, starting at the base of the neck, then working outward across the top of the shoulders. Repeat two or three times, then interlace your fingers at the back of the neck and squeeze the heels of the hands together to make a delicious clamp for tired neck and shoulder muscles. (You can also use this technique on his upper arm muscles.) Use your hands to squeeze and relax the muscles repeatedly across the neck and shoulders. As a finishing touch lightly sweep the hands in gliding motions over the whole region.

Shoulder rolling Kneel behind your partner with your feet raised and flexed and place your forearms on his shoulders, directly against the base of the neck. Your hands should be relaxed, with palms facing downward. Lean slightly forward, allowing your body weight to place pressure onto the trapezius muscles, then roll your forearms outward along the muscles to just before the shoulder bones – your palms should now be facing upward. Roll the arms back again, then repeat the technique two or three times.

Thai bodywork 85

Butterfly postures

These beautiful butterfly postures are balletic to watch and help to loosen up the shoulder blades and the muscles of the torso. Beware of stretching the arms too far – men's muscles in particular may be tight, so work slowly and carefully.

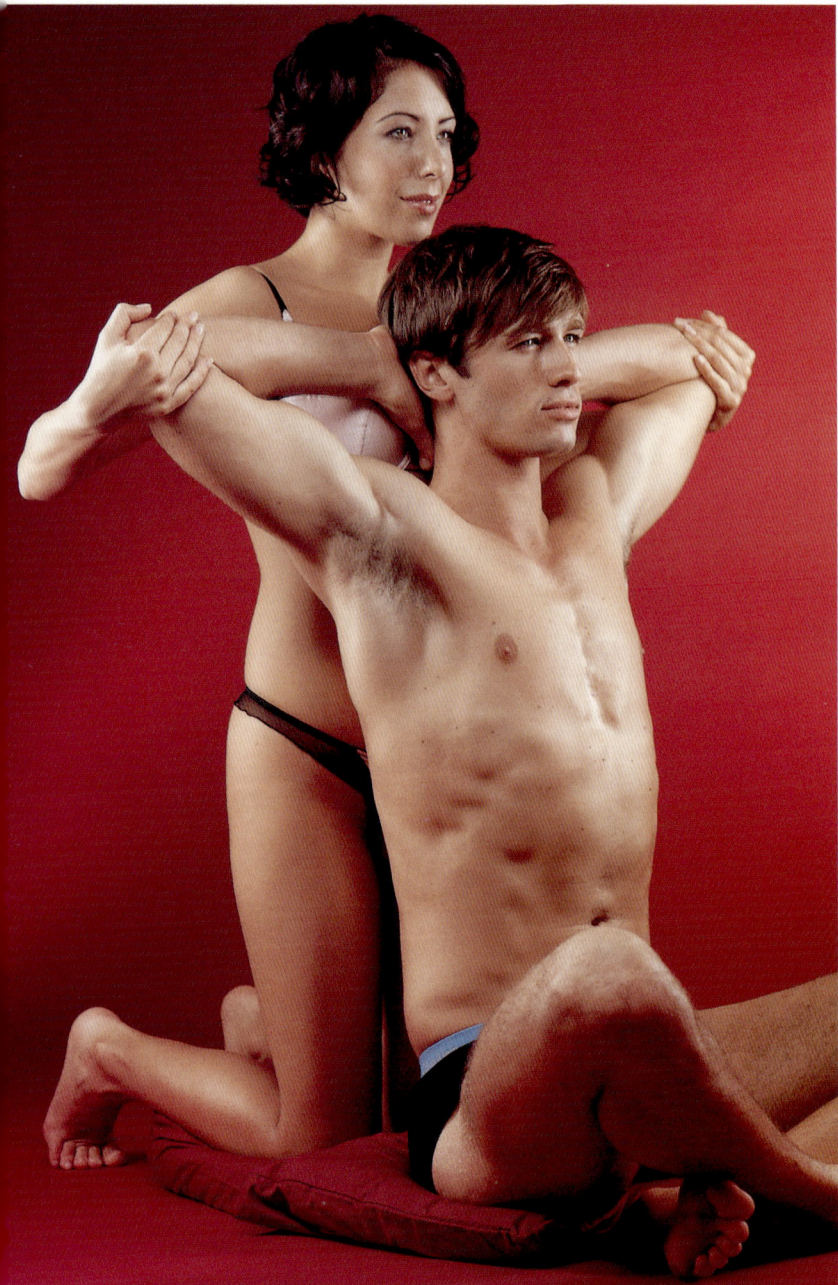

1 Butterfly wing stretch Ask your partner to interlace the fingers behind his neck. Take his elbows in your hands. Hold for a little while so he can warm and adjust to the opening of the rib cage and chest and straightening of the spine. Cradle your partner into your body so its warmth helps the muscles to relax. Make your beloved feel nurtured and unhurried with your touch, matching the pattern of his breathing. When you are both ready, hold the elbows and ease your body farther into your partner's back and lever the elbows farther backward to gently increase the pressure of the stretch. Release on a long out-breath and hold gently. Repeat two or three times at leisure.

Hot tip
With all Thai bodywork postures, make sure that you work only on muscles that have been gently stretched beforehand or warmed up in a bath or shower. Never attempt the twists with people who have bad back problems.

Butterfly twist Weave your forearms under and around your partner's upper arms, placing your hands on his wrists or your interlaced fingers onto the back of his neck, or even keep the previous handhold on the elbows. Create a stable framework for your body by placing your right foot flat on the floor beside your partner and resting your weight on your left heel. By pressing your body closely to your partner's torso you will ensure that he maintains an upright and uplifted alignment at all times. Wait until your partner inhales and, matching his exhalation, twist his entire upper torso to the right using your stance as a lever. Your left knee will drop on to your partner's left thigh, stabilizing his pelvis and ensuring a safe and controlled twist. Inhale and fully release the stretch, returning to the central position. Take a few natural breaths before repeating the twist sequence two or three more times, then change your supporting legs and twist to the left two or three times. Work as strongly or as gently as your partner's body clearly allows.

Butterfly side stretch Position yourself at your partner's left side with your knee anchored firmly on his thigh. Rest your weight on your raised, arched left foot. Your right knee is by the left hip, with shin and foot flat on the floor. Place your partner's left palm against the left side of his head, with the heel of the hand pressed lightly against the temple and fingers molding gently around the top of the head. Support the left elbow with your right hand and place your left hand on the right shoulder to keep the position square. Inhale, then exhale and push the left elbow away from you, creating a long stretch down the left side. Your partner's right hand can be placed on your knee. It's important to remember that your partner's body is only stretched sideways, not twisted. When your partner is ready to inhale, release the stretch and allow him to straighten up. Repeat two or three times, holding him in the final stretched position for as long as is comfortable. Repeat two or three times on the other side to balance the body.

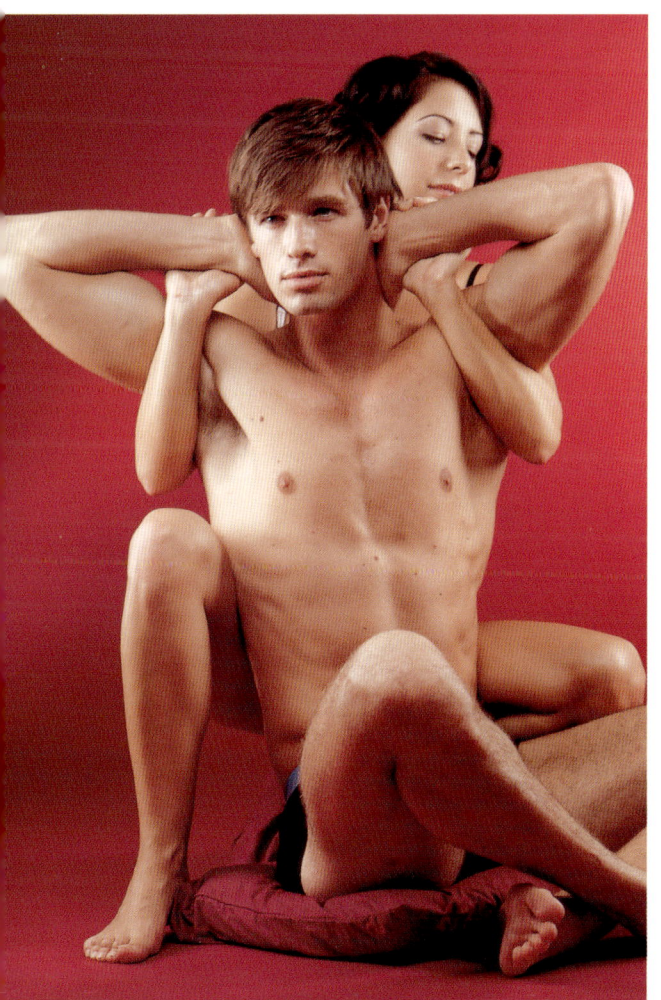
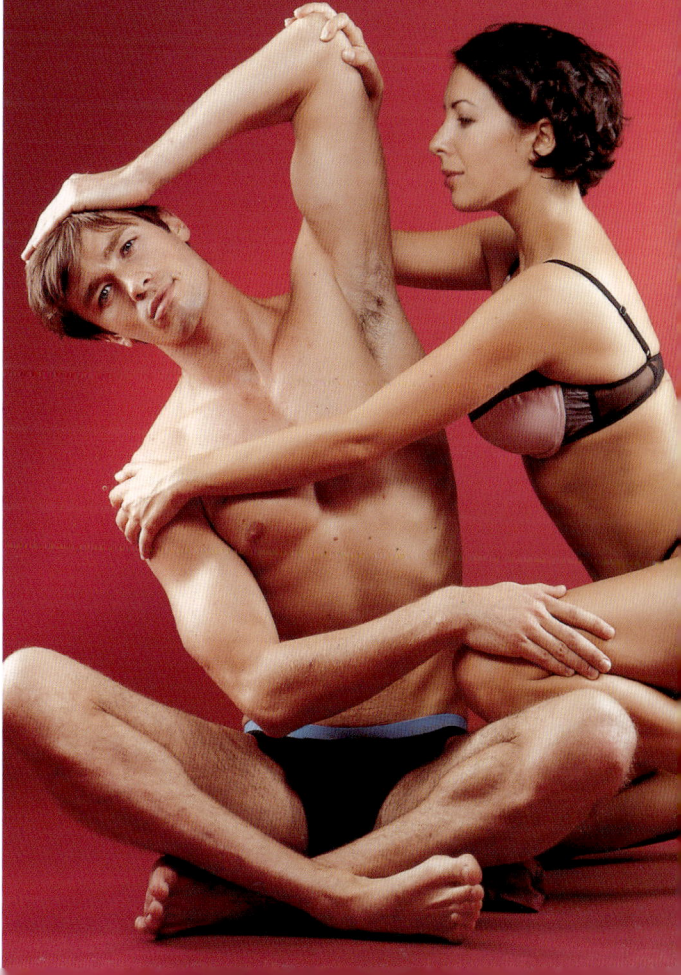

Hot seat cobra

This sequence involves an important back bend that is found in all bodywork and movement systems, from yoga to martial arts and Thai bodywork. Imitating the posture of an aroused cobra, it provides a strong and vitalizing stretch for the lower back. Since its successful application relies on careful leverage and balance, it's possible for a slight woman to position even a heavily muscled man in a strong stretch.

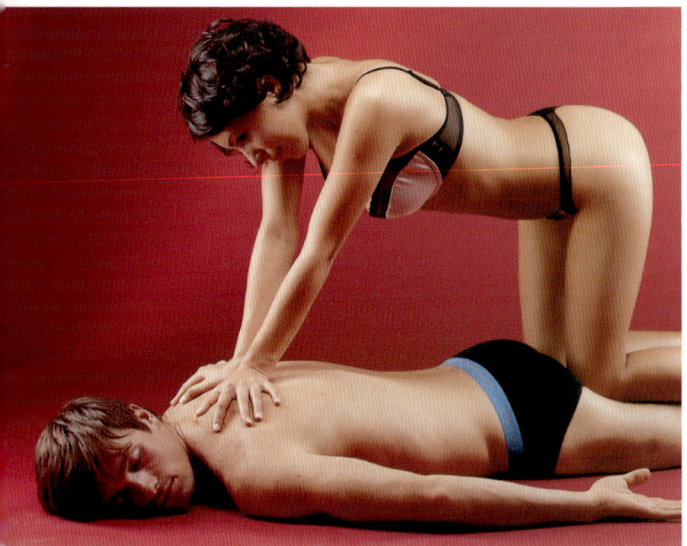 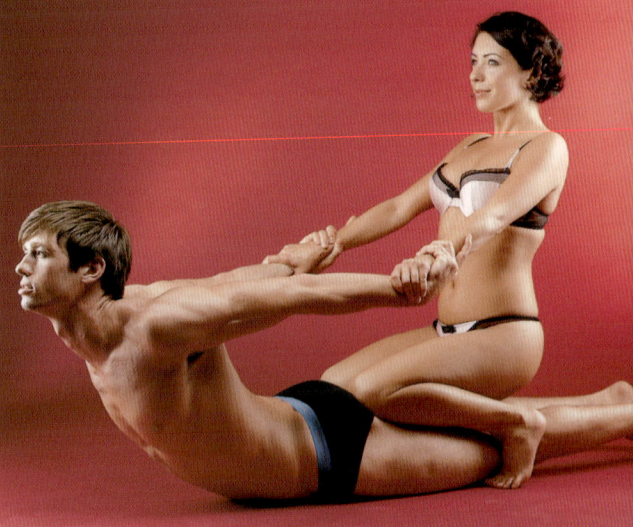

Back press Ask your partner to lie flat on the massage surface with palms facing upward. Position yourself either with your legs balanced on the backs of the thighs and calves with your knees positioned near the buttocks, or kneeling astride your partner. With your body adopting a four-square cat position, place the heel of your hands on the muscles to either side of the spine at the level of the shoulder blades. Once your breathing is synchronized with your partner's, lean your body weight down onto the back on an exhalation. Inhale in time with your partner's natural inhalation, reposition your hands a little way down and press down with your body weight as you both exhale. Continue down the spine to the mid-back. Proceed up and down the back as many times as you wish.

Striking cobra Now grasp one another's wrists. Exhale, then inhale together as you lean back, using your weight to lift your partner's upper body into a cobra position. Your toes should be flexed and placed on the floor on either side of your partner's legs to take some of the weight. As you are maintaining the position, your partner can keep his head, neck and shoulder muscles relaxed in a natural curve. Ask him to contract the buttock muscles and shoulder blades. Breathe lightly as you both give in to the stretch, ensuring that your eyes are focused on a point straight ahead of you. Ensure your partner does not overarch the head, which could cause tension in the neck. Release the arms and allow your partner to relax into the floor.

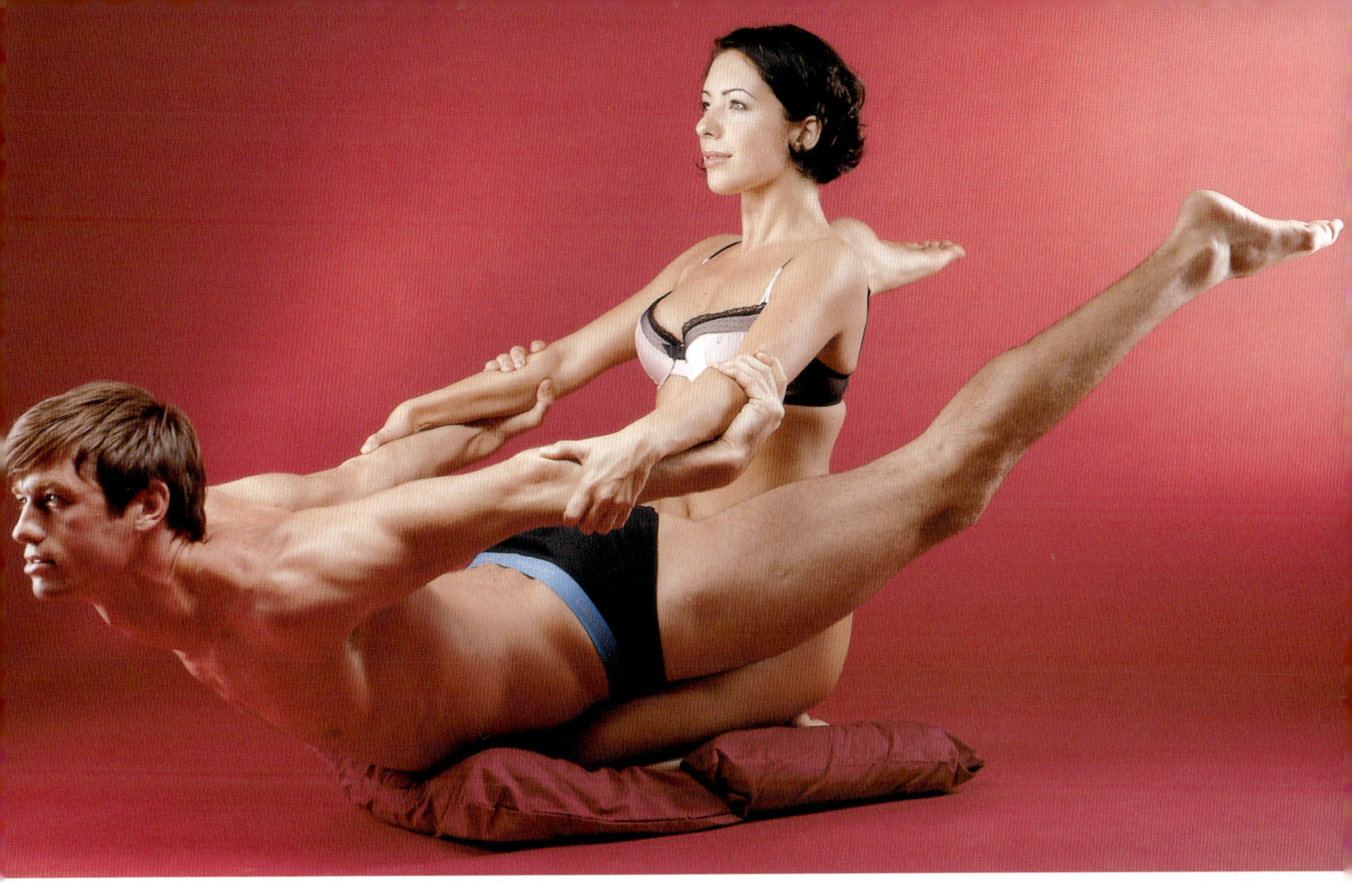

Flying cobra Ask your partner to raise his hips as you slide your thighs between the legs and raise your partner's thighs and hips onto yours. You may choose to use a cushion to make this position more comfortable for your partner. Lean forward and take the elbows in a secure grip. Exhale, then inhale together as you lean backward to facilitate another cobra lift and stretch. Your partner should assist by contracting the shoulder blades and buttocks to lift the legs while the head, neck and shoulder muscles remain as relaxed as possible. This step is a balancing act in more ways than one, as you both need to exercise control and relaxation at the same time. Hold the pose for a few gentle breaths, then exhale as you gently ease down and out of the position in a controlled manner. Repeat two to three times.

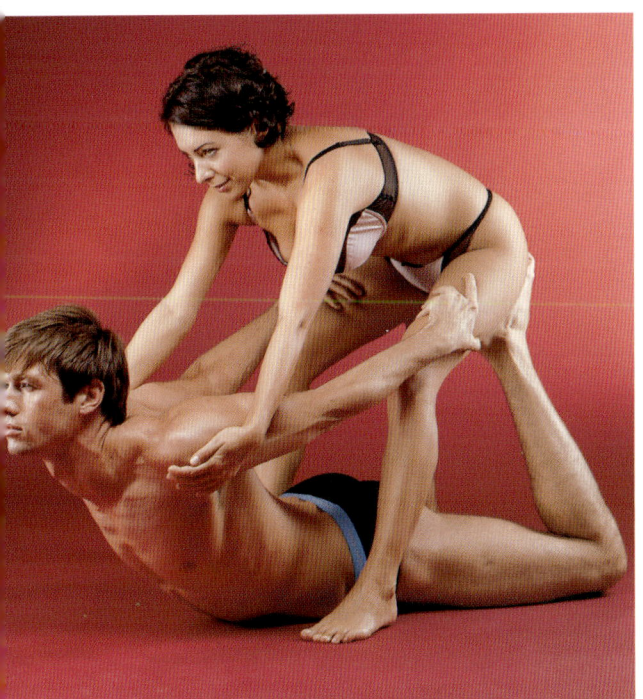

Hot seat cobra Ask your partner to raise the lower legs so that the feet form a comfortable seat for you. Place your buttocks on the seat with your feet positioned on either side of your partner's waist or hips. Lean forward and cup your partner's shoulder bones. Your partner should reach back and clasp your thighs or calves – wherever is most comfortable. Once again, exhale then inhale as you pull the shoulders back, using the strength of your thigh muscles – not your back muscles – to raise his upper torso from the floor into the cobra position. Hold for a few gentle breaths, then slowly lower the position with control. Repeat two or three times.

Statuesque stretches

This series of stretches bring your Thai bodywork session to a close. It is important to end with these stretches as the muscles will contract after the exertion of the sequence shown in this chapter, making them more susceptible to injury. By stretching the muscles directly after exercise, you help prevent injury, reduce stiffness and improve your flexibility.

1 Body stretch Ask your partner to sit cross-legged or, if preferable, with knees bent and feet flat on the floor. Sit behind your partner, on a cushion or pillow if desired, with knees bent and calves and feet tucked under you, bringing your knees close to her lower back. Position a pillow on your thighs and ask your partner to lean back, stretch her arms up and place her palms on your shoulders or, if more comfortable, interlace her fingers behind your neck. Gently clasp her hands for additional support. Exhale, then inhale as you lean back as far as you're both able to, creating a delicious body stretch. Hold, breathing gently for a few breaths, then inhale and, with control, straighten up. Repeat the move, synchronized with the breath, two or three times.

2 Assisted arch Adjust your position so that you are sitting with knees raised, feet flat on the floor and toes beneath your partner's buttocks. Your shins and knees, covered with a pillow, provide a backrest for your partner, who should sit either cross-legged in front of you or with knees bent and feet flat on the floor. This time, clasp under your partner's upper arms, close to the armpits as she clasps your biceps or shoulders. Exhale, then inhale as you lean back creating a lengthening stretch in your partner's back. Hold the pose, breathing gently for a few breaths, then exhale as you release the position. Repeat two or three times. As a variation, when you are in the final stretched position, rock from side to side to deepen the stretch and lengthen the spine with a gentle traction.

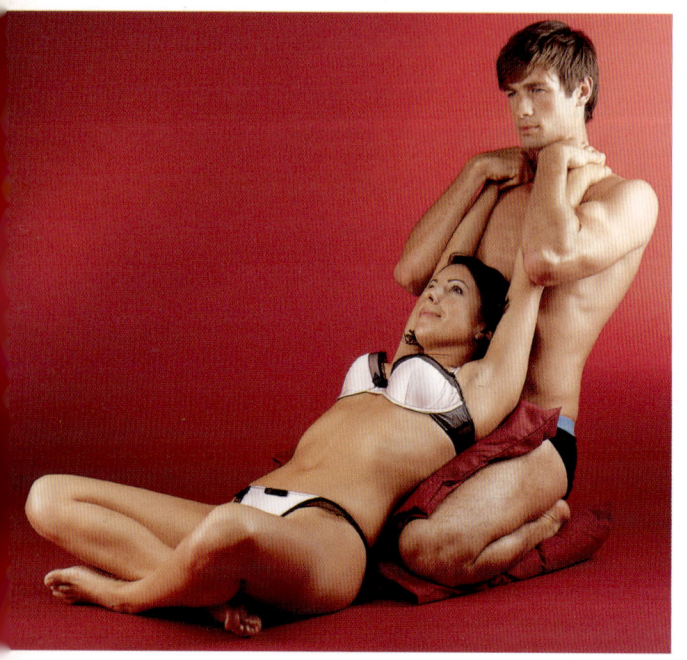
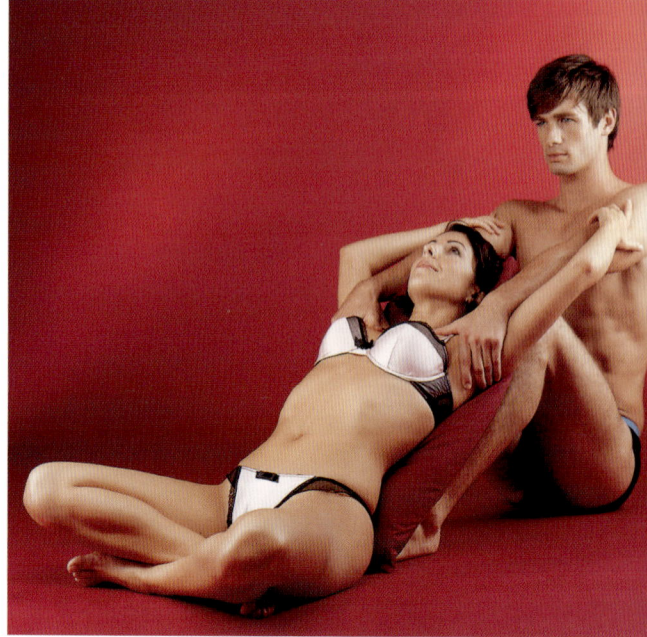

Supported bridge Ask your partner to sit with knees bent and feet and knees hip-width apart. Sit behind her, with knees bent and feet flat on the floor. Place a cushion on your knees and ask her to lean back against your shins and knees. With your partner holding your biceps and your hands clasping her shoulders, exhale together, then inhale and lean backward, bringing your body to the floor. As you do this, your partner pushes up with her legs and you ease her into position with the small of her back resting on your knees, forming a bridge shape. Hold the posture, breathing gently, then exhale and release in a controlled manner. Take a few natural breaths and repeat two or three times.

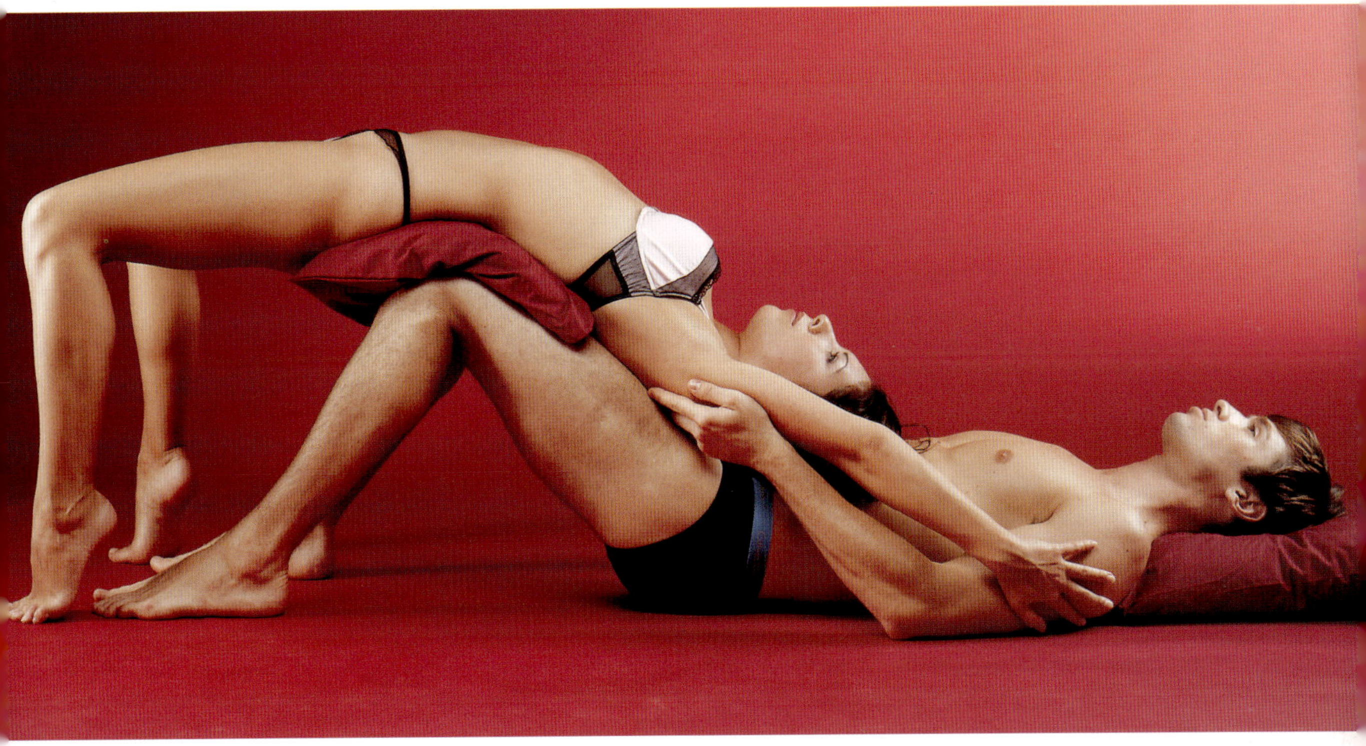

Body wrap As a counterpoise, sit cross-legged before each other with knees touching. Ask your partner to bend forward into your lap, head on one of your thighs. Now bend forward and mold yourself around your partner's back. Relax and breathe gently together. The body wrap provides a peaceful finishing touch to your Thai bodywork session.

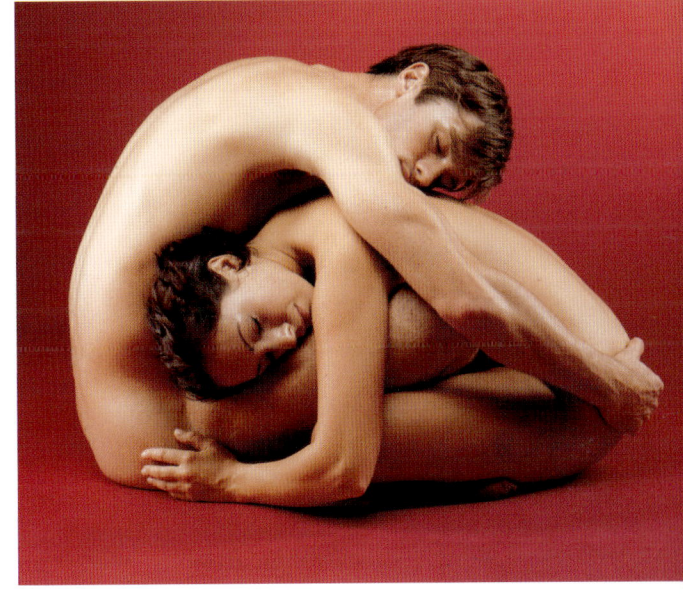

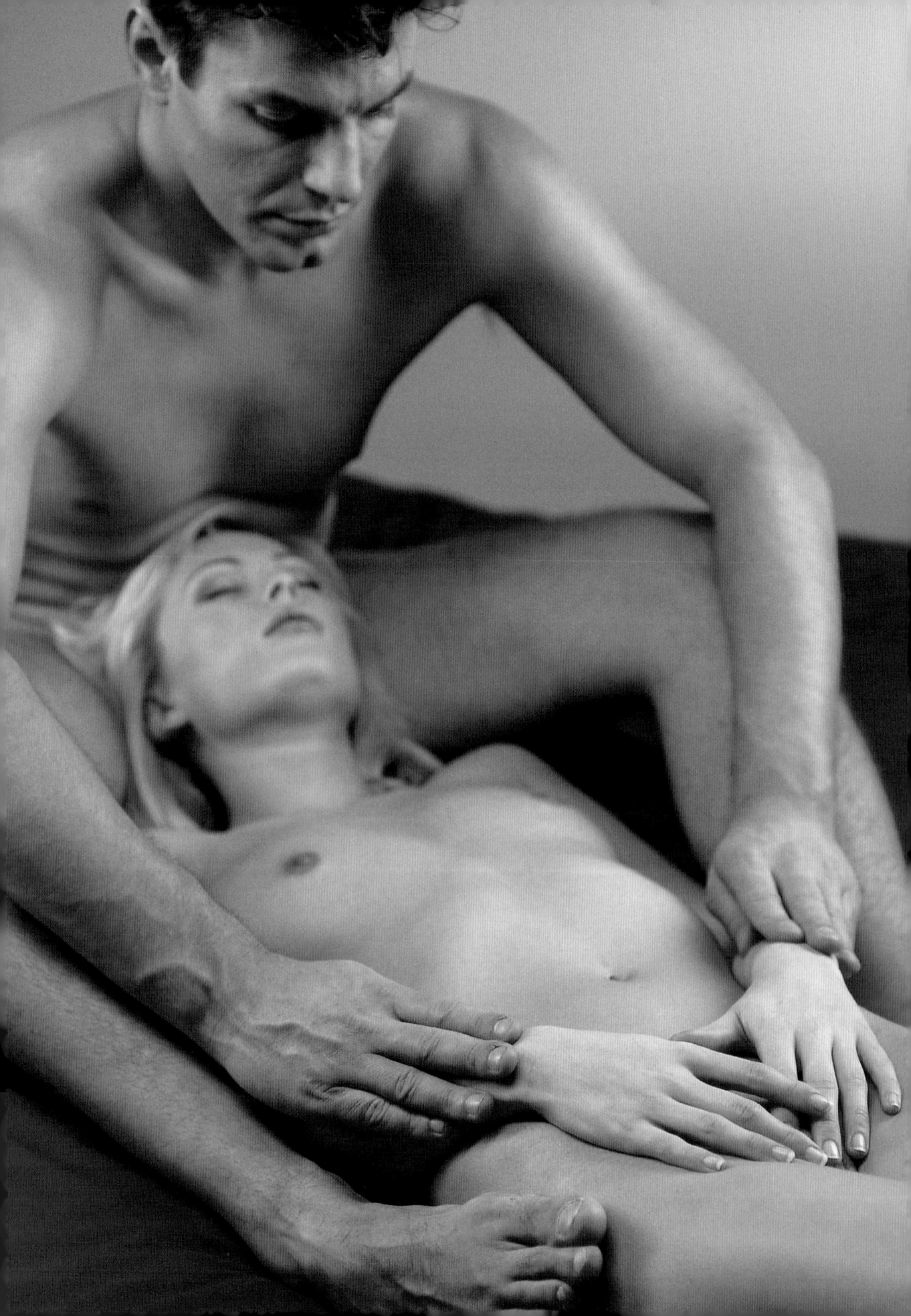

Top to toe

Connect to and awaken every part of your partner's body with the following complete head-to-toe massage sequence.

The head and face

This chapter offers a complete massage sequence, working down the body from head to feet, developing from gentle to deep pressure. The sequence is easy to follow and you can develop it in your own special way. Ask your partner to lie down on the floor on her back, with hands resting on the body and with cushions supporting the head and the backs of the knees. During the massage, keep looking at your partner's face for signs of feedback.

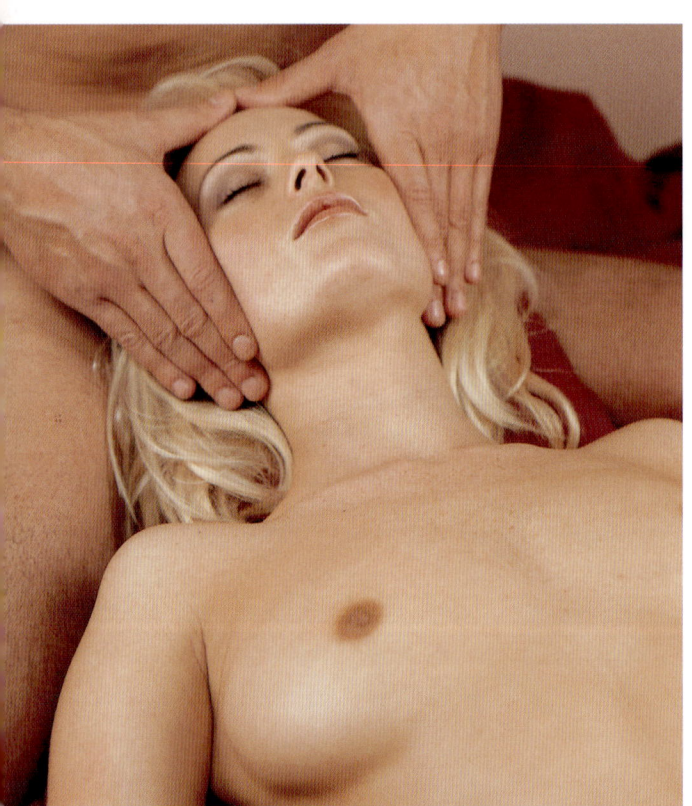

1 Face smoothing Sit behind your partner's head and place both thumbs on the forehead along the hairline, with your fingers framing the face. Pressing evenly with the pads of the thumbs, glide the thumbs out across and around the hairline to the depressions in the sides of the temples. Trail back and return to a point just below the starting position, a little farther down the forehead, and repeat, gradually covering the whole of the forehead down to a point between the eyebrows. Now position the thumbs at the base of the bridge of the nose, under the corner of the eyes, and gently glide them out along the bony part of the eye sockets to the temples. Return the thumbs to a point a little below the starting position and repeat until the whole of the cheeks have been smoothed out. As you smooth over the lines of worry on the face, imagine each touch is erasing away the tension that builds up under the skin and deepens these lines.

Hot tip
As a finishing touch, cup your hands over your partner's ears and pause for a few minutes before continuing with the massage.

2 Chin pressing Press into a point below the center of the lower lip on the chin bone and continue out along the chin bone toward the temples. Repeat, pressing the chin between the thumb and index fingers along the edge of the jaw and finish by circling three times with the middle fingertips on the temples.

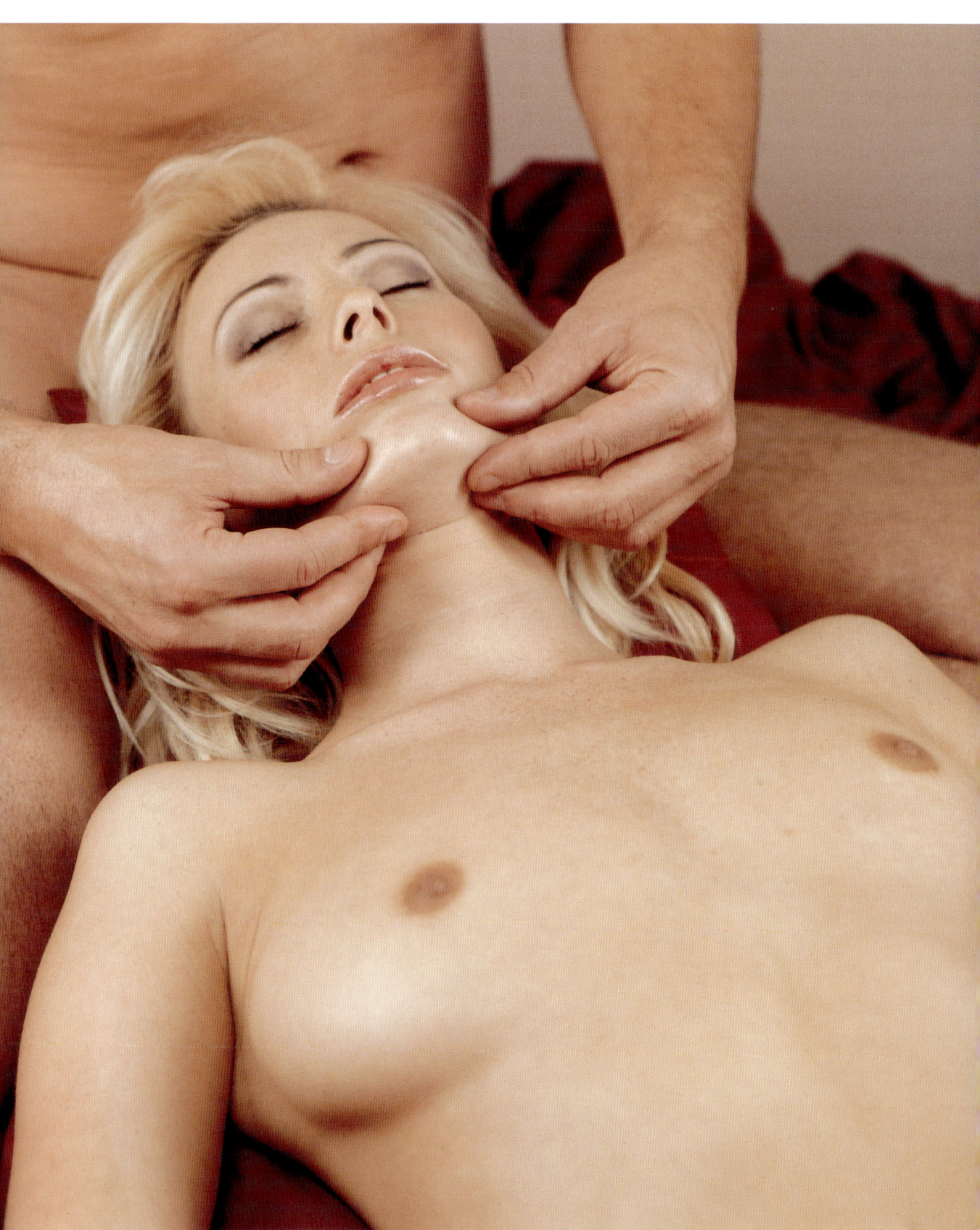

Neck and shoulders

It is quite commonplace for us to hold the stresses and strains of our worldly pressures in our neck and shoulders, and so many of us spend hours each day sitting at desks in front of computers, which can also create tension in this region. The following steps will help to relieve such tension. For this section of the massage remain seated behind your partner's head. Her head should be between your legs and cushions should be used to support the head and the backs of the knees.

Rest your hands over the tops of your partner's shoulders and push them down in the direction of the feet with a firm and steady pressure. Hold for five to ten seconds. Release slightly and repeat the movement three times.

Place your hands over the shoulders, with the heels against the trapezius muscles and the fingers resting on the upper parts of the chest so that the hands form a triangle. Press down firmly and hold for five to ten seconds. Release and repeat three times.

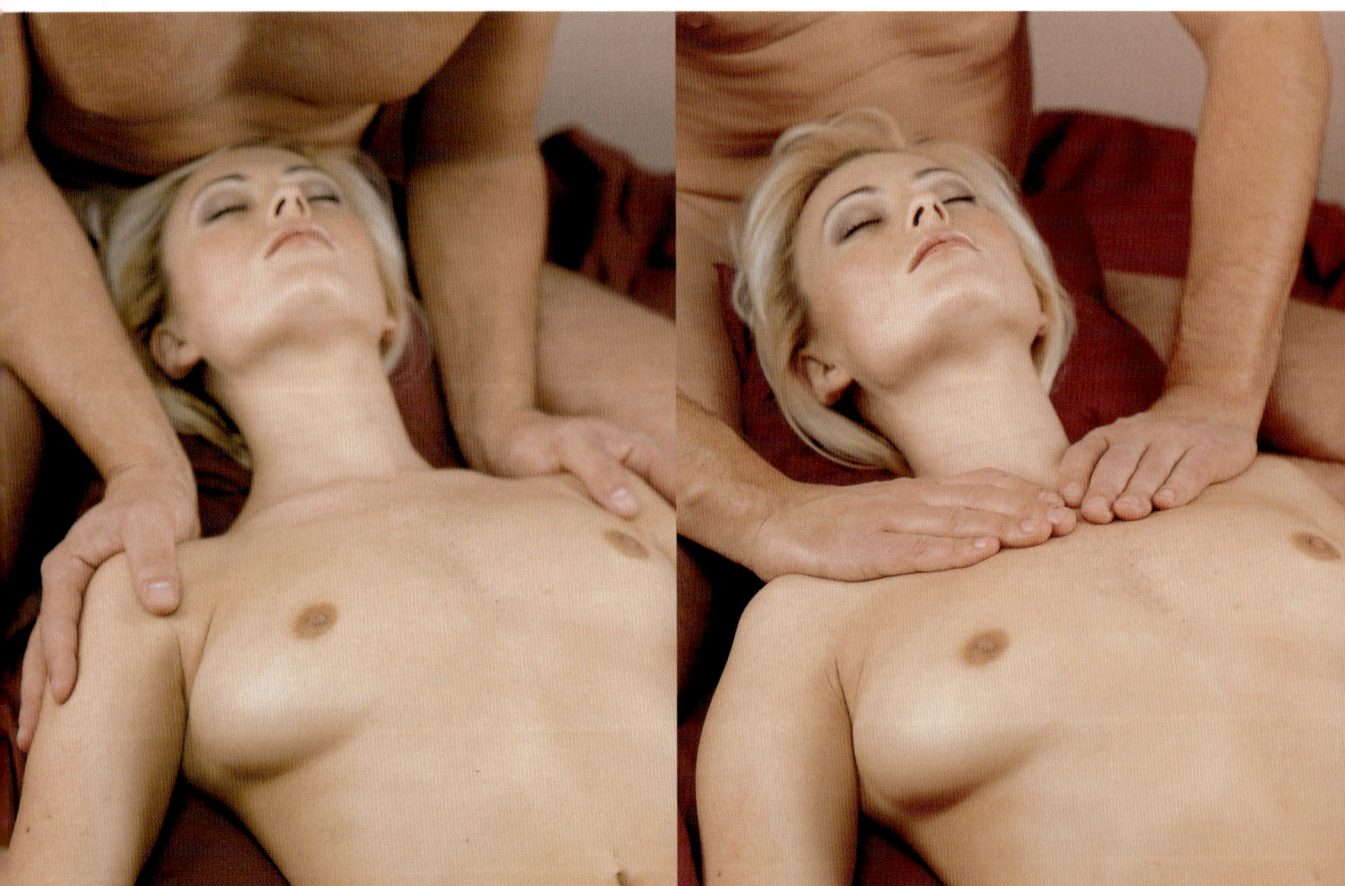

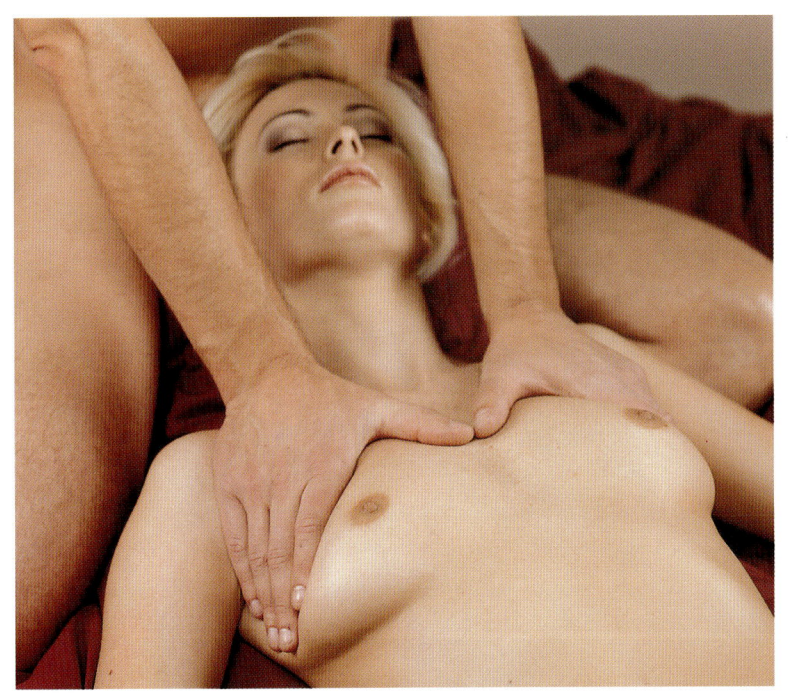

3 Glide your hands outward across the chest and rest them on the upper part of the chest. Press firmly down into the floor to help open the upper chest. Release slightly and repeat the movement three times.

4 Slide your hands under your partner's shoulder blades, spreading your fingers like flattened claws. Assist your partner to arch the back slightly as you rake your hands up the body and neck. Repeat two or three times. Finish by tailing off with your fingers gently at the back of the head.

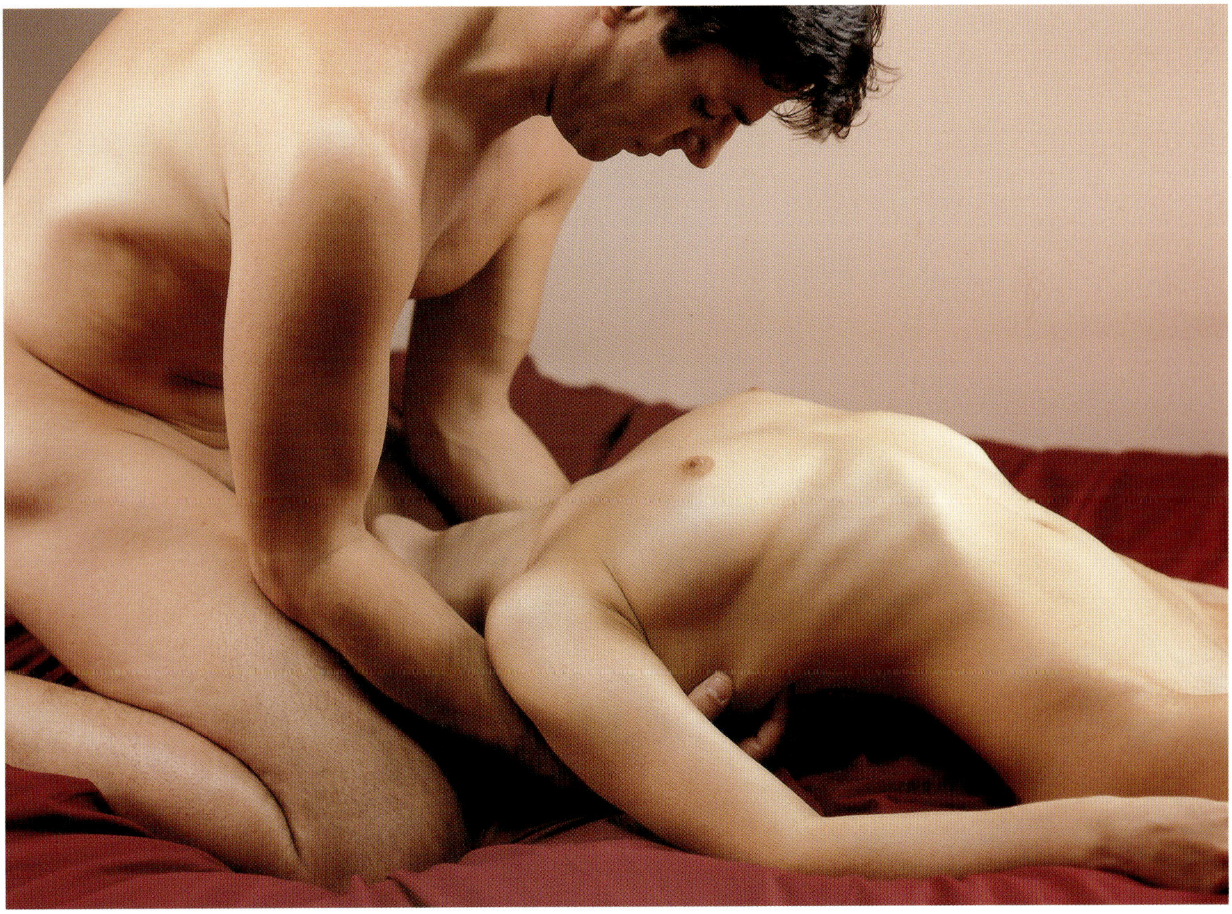

The arms

Massaging the arms can bring astonishingly strong waves of relief, as much more tension is held in the arms than is often expected. The sensation can be highly arousing. Remain in position, seated behind your partner's head, and nestle the soles of your feet into the side of your partner's rib cage or waist for support and leverage.

Streamlining Using your working hand, take hold of one of your partner's arms by the back of the wrist or the forearm. As you inhale, gently extend the arm back and into the side of your body, securing it with your supporting hand. Hold momentarily then ease the arm slightly out of its stretch on the out-breath. Relax momentarily before inhaling again as you repeat the stretching process two to three times, synchronized with your inhalations. Lower the arm back down onto the body and repeat with the other arm. Then repeat the whole sequence two or three times with both arms.

As a finishing touch, lean forward and lower your partner's hands onto the abdomen, then glide your hands in one long continuous, smooth stroke along the hands, arms, shoulders, the back of the neck and up behind the ears, then rake your fingertips gently through the scalp. Stroke the hairline to finish.

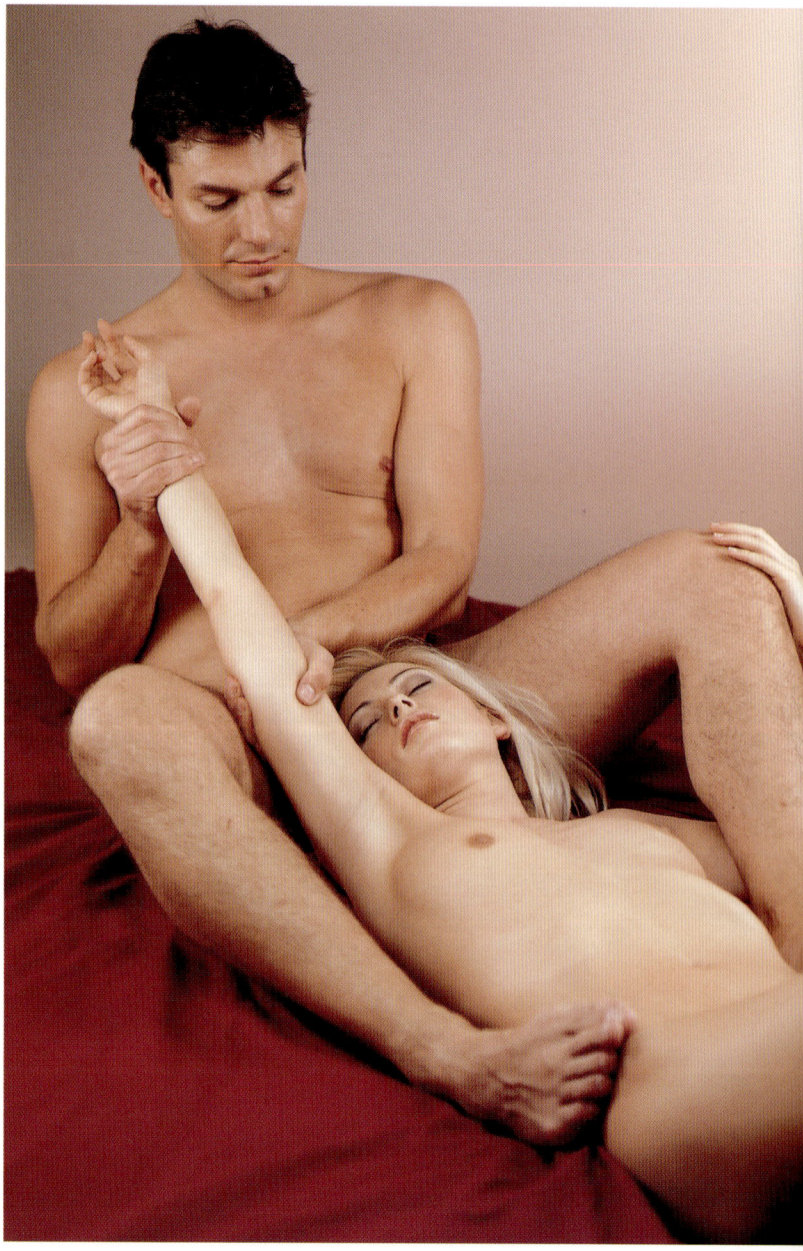

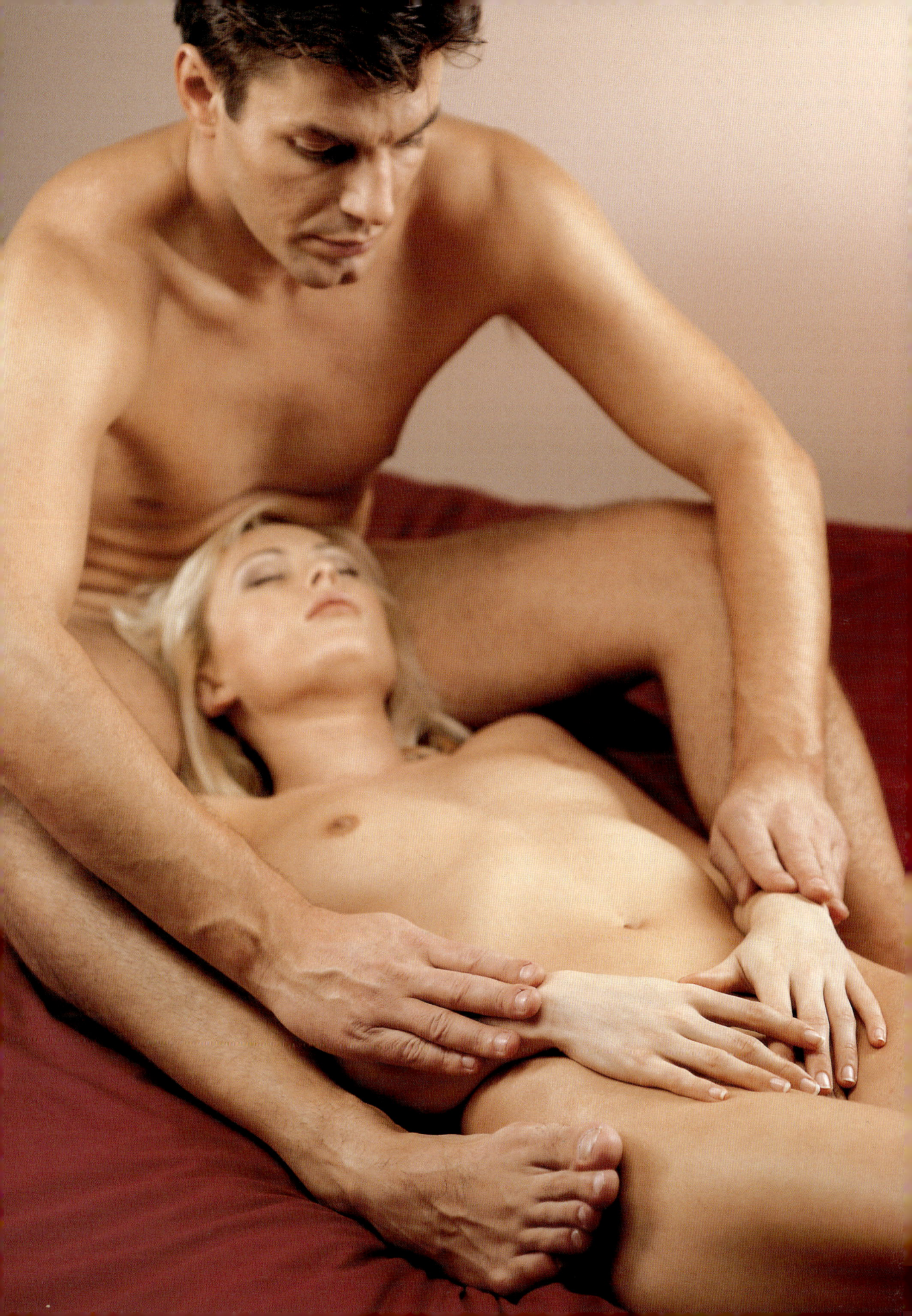

The torso

This technique is a fluid, crossover, figure eight style movement, reminiscent of a spring flowing through a boulder-strewn watercourse. You can perform it either with lotion, talc or oil on a naked body or over smooth, silky clothing. It is simple and nurturing, with the benefit of easing neck and shoulder tensions. During the sequence, the hands graze the breasts and groin, which connects these pleasure zones to the rest of the body's sensations. Kneel beside your partner's left side, facing her head and shoulders to perform this "flowing spring" movement.

1 Cross your arms over your partner's chest and gently clasp the neck and shoulder muscles. Maintaining a natural rhythm of breathing throughout, open your elbows as you slide your arms down the body, drawing on the muscles, and bring your hands to meet at the level of the heart, one over another.

2 Keeping the hands connected by resting one hand on top of the other or interweaving the fingers, continue the gliding action in a fluid movement, around and under the right rib cage to grip the right side of the waist momentarily and ease the muscle away from the spine.

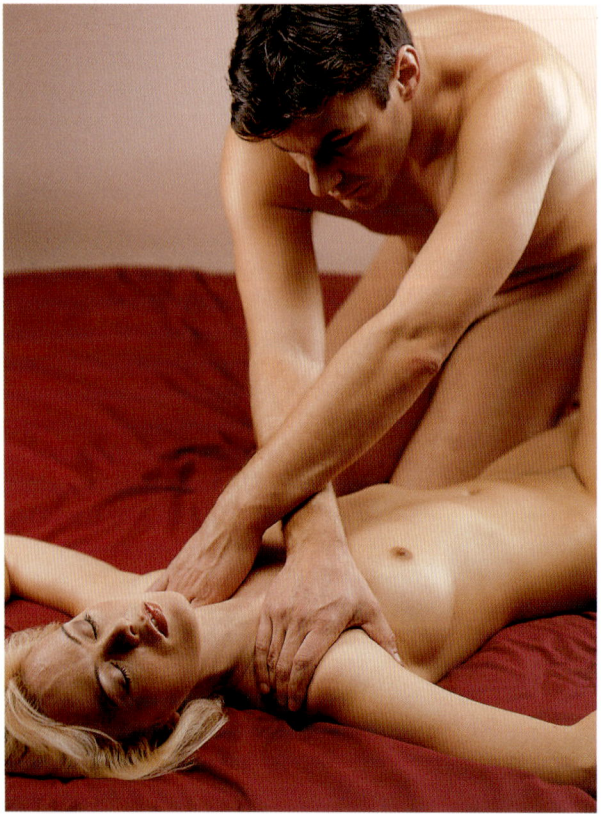
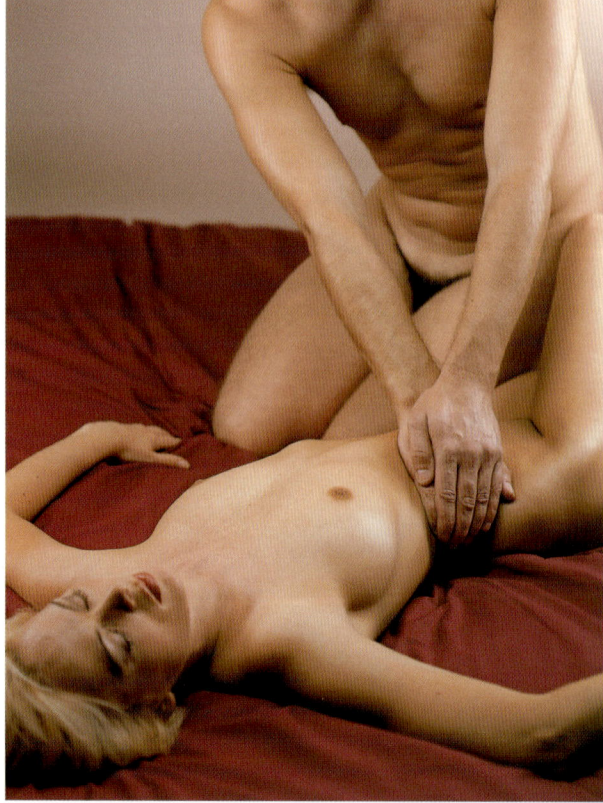

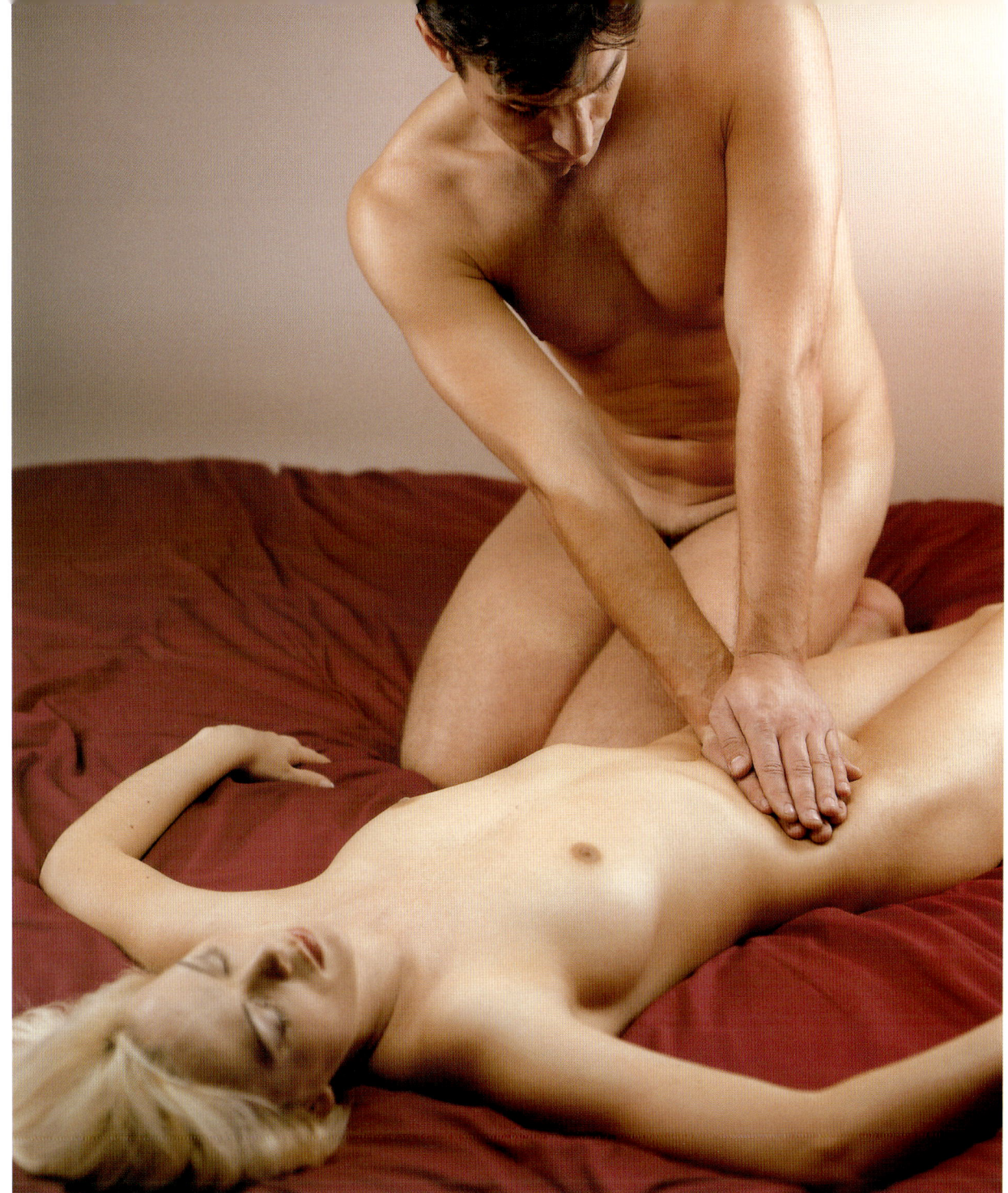

Continue the flowing movement with the butt of the lower hand, gliding it onto the groin, lightly brushing the genitals, then moving up to hook momentarily around the left side of the waist. The movement continues back to the heart, the hands and arms once again crossing at the chest to clasp the neck and shoulder muscles. Ensure you keep a flowing rhythm linked to your breathing.

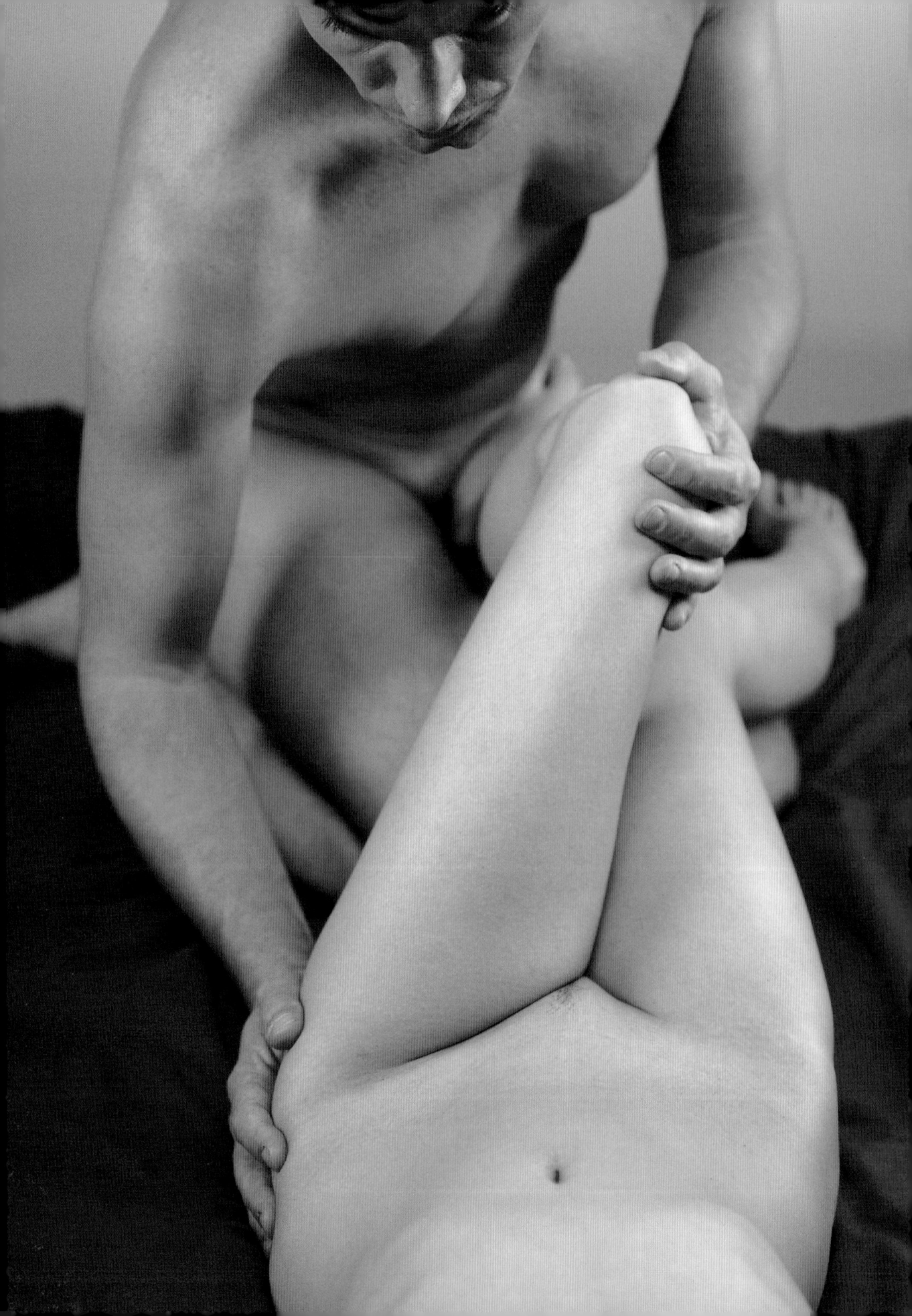

Thighs and genitals

These tantalizers will excite your partner as well as yourself and you make contact with her genitals as part of the massage. From your position beside your partner's left side, move farther down the body to kneel or sit cross-legged beside the left knee, then bend your partner's knees and position the left foot in your lap. Ensure that one hand or another always supports the knee in the upright position to enable your partner to feel totally relaxed.

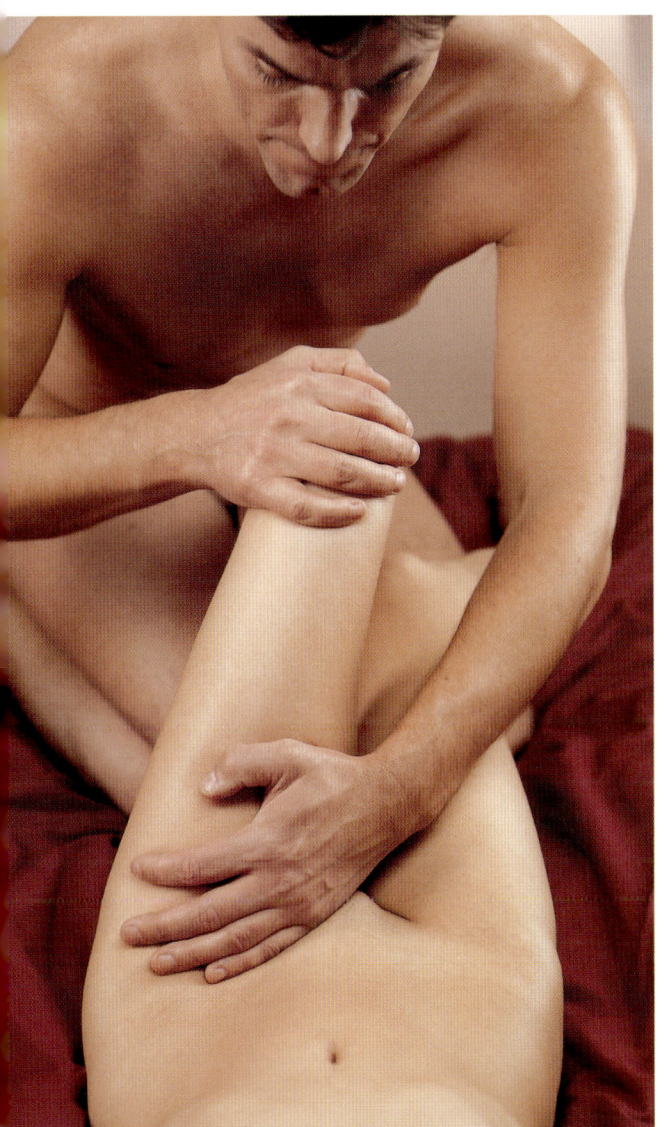

1 **With your left hand cupping** and supporting the knee, smooth the whole of your right hand down along the outer edge of the thigh and round the hip. Hook under the buttock, then trail the hand along the buttock crease. Then lightly brush the genitals or vulva before gliding the hand up the back and inner thigh to the back of the knee.

2 **Now replace** the left hand with the right and allow it to perform a similar stroke, gliding the palm down the front of the thigh into the crease between leg and groin, again lightly brushing the genitals and flowing up the inner thigh to the back of the knee. Repeat the sequence as often as you wish. Straighten out the left leg, shift your position slightly over to the right, lift the right leg and place the foot in your lap. Now repeat steps 1 and 2, reversing the hand positions.

lightly brush the genitals or vulva before **gliding** the hand up the back and **inner thigh**

Lower legs

For these strokes, move to the right side of your partner's body and sit in a cross-legged or kneeling position, making a resting place for her legs so the knee of the bent left leg rests over your thigh and the left foot is placed on it. This position will help to relieve any tension in your partner's lower back. She may either lie flat on her back, or raised and supported by cushions or her elbows, in order to feel part of the action.

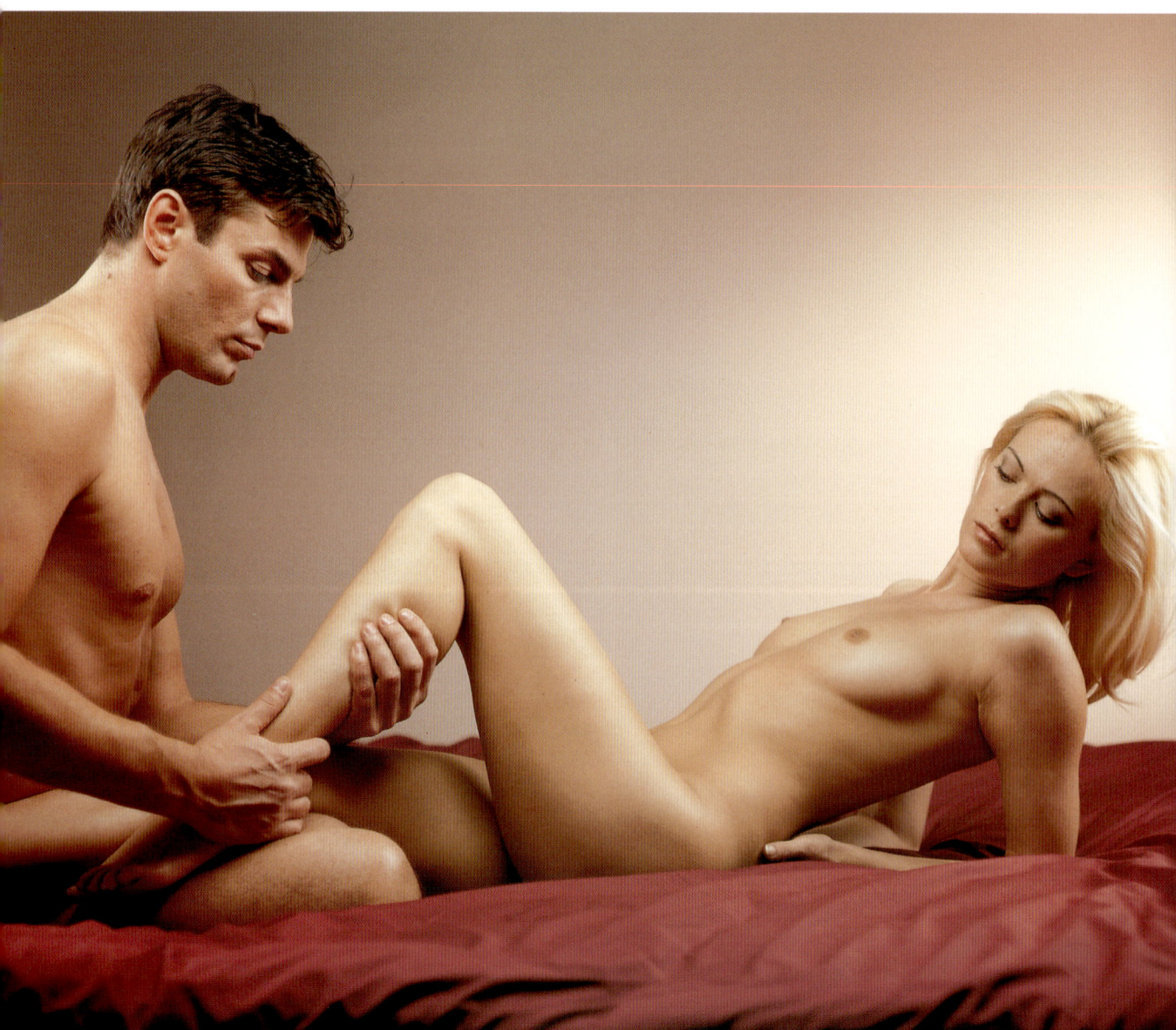

Squeeze around the ankle bone and Achilles tendon with both hands. Now anchor the foot to your thigh with your right hand and use your left hand to squeeze and release the calf muscle, working from the Achilles tendon to the knee and back again. Smooth off with simple soothing strokes, then repeat as many times as you wish. Circle the kneecap with your left hand, then stroke down along the shin and smooth off through the top of the foot. Circle around the base of the toes on the top of the foot with the palm of your hand. Repeat three or four times.

Support the knee with your left hand to keep it upright, and use your right hand to stroke the top of the foot and gently squeeze the metatarsal bones above and between the toes. Grasp the toes firmly in your fist and gently bend them in both directions of flexion. Pull each toe gently in turn and repeat the whole sequence. Since so many nerves (both subtle and physical) terminate in the foot, massaging and flexing the foot can initiate twinges and sensations in seemingly unrelated parts of the body. Repeat steps 1 and 2 on the right leg and foot.

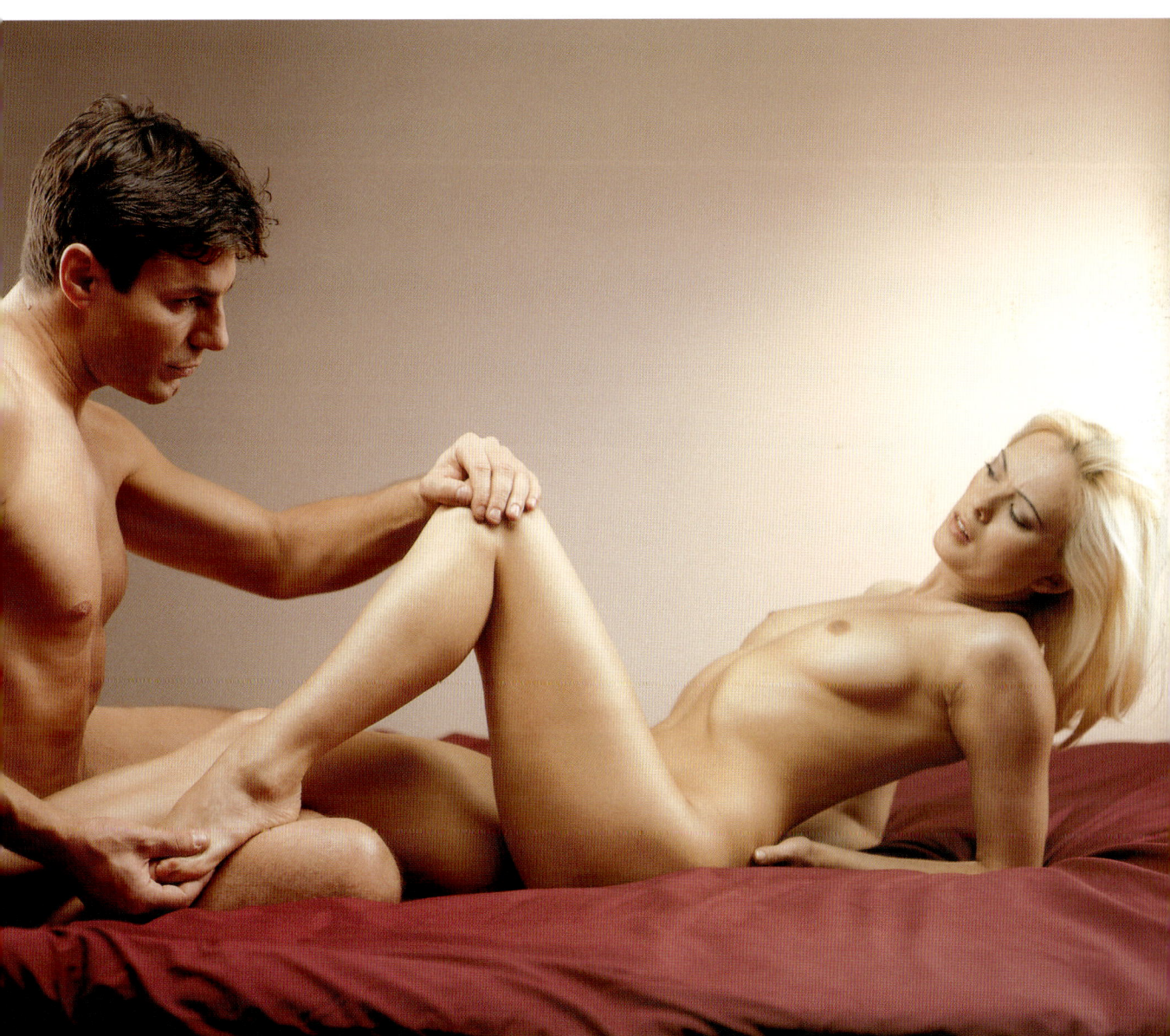

Spine: Awakening twist

This is one of the most important sections of the book as far as overall benefits are concerned. The spine is home to our nervous system. Lengthening and stretching the outer and inner deep-seated muscles and easing and aligning the vertebrae can have immediate beneficial results.

Still seated beneath your partner's right hip, bend her knees up so that her feet are flat on the floor near the buttocks. Assist the instep of the right foot onto the left knee as you pull the left foot toward you so that the left knee and thigh are in line with the torso and the right knee crosses the body. This creates a delicious cross stretch that relieves back muscles, leaving your partner's body free for a range of massage strokes. If your partner is willing and able, assist her to grasp the left foot with the right hand, ensuring that the right shoulder remains as close to the floor as possible. The head should be turned the opposite way to the stretch so your partner should be looking over her right shoulder. Until she gets used to the position and learns to relax, help your partner by placing helping hands on her right shoulder and right hip. The placement of cushions or pillows should be enough to make this position comfortable even for the stiffest of bodies. It is not crucial that the fullest stretch be obtained or maintained.

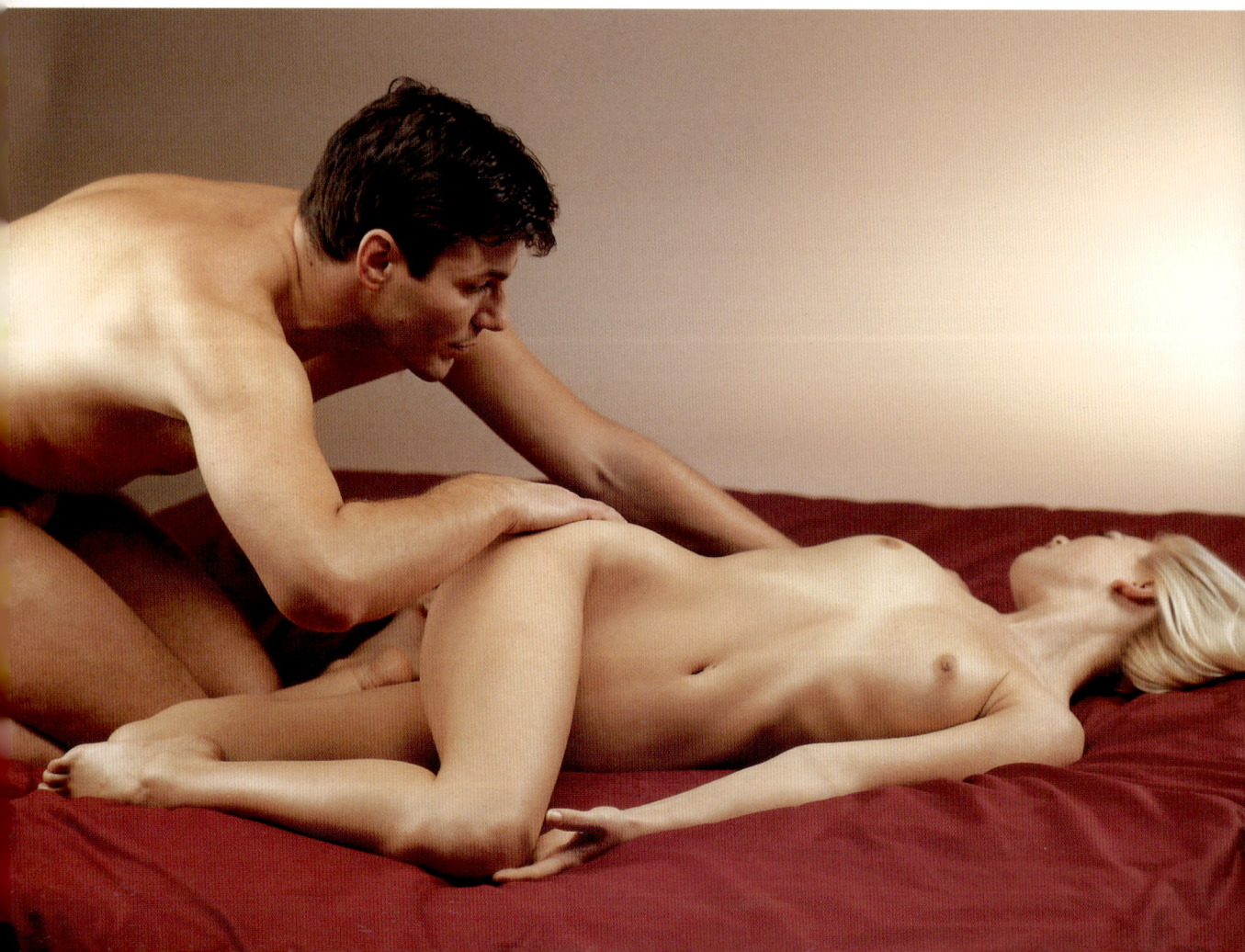

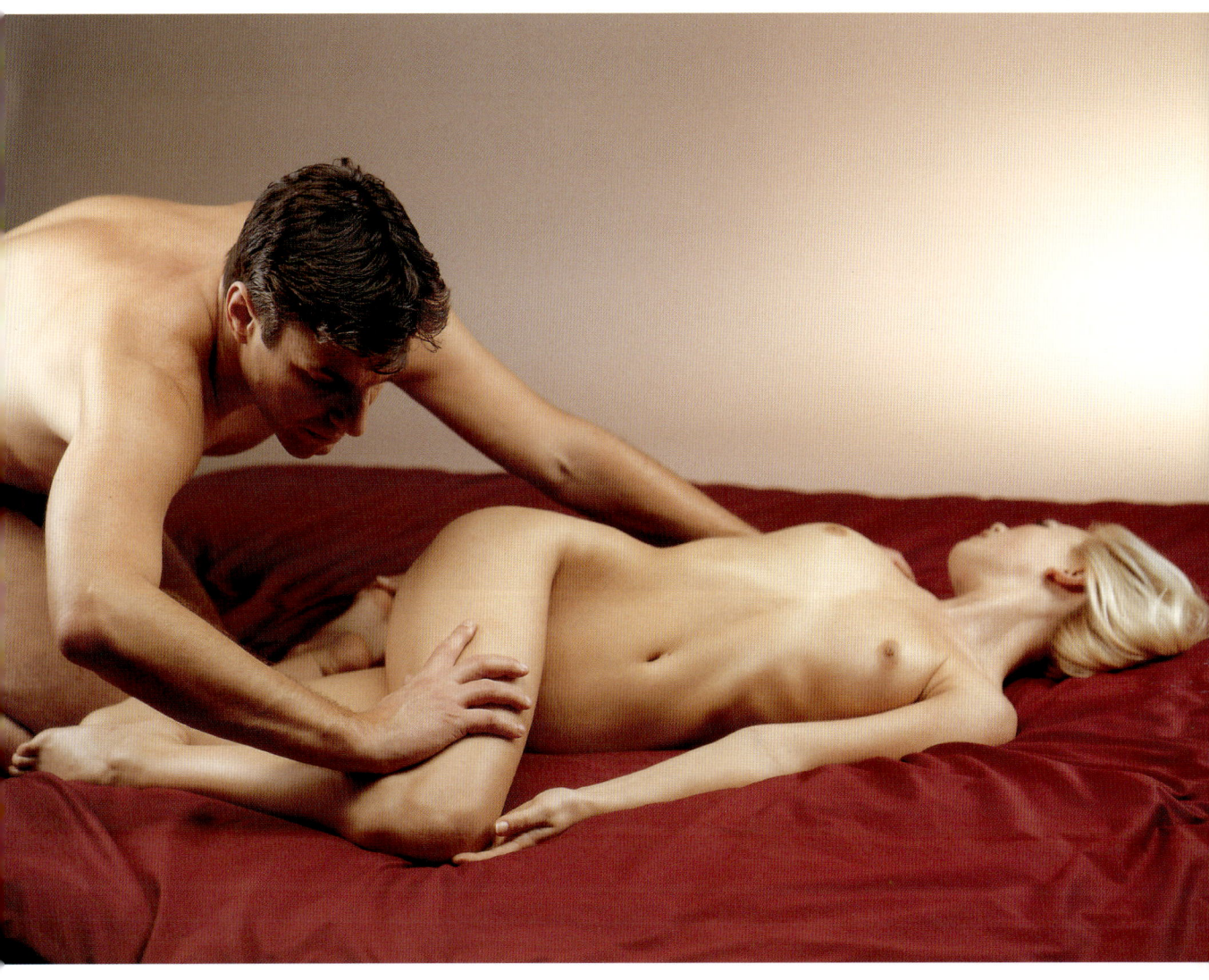

a **delicious** cross stretch that **relieves** back muscles, leaving your partner's body **free** for a range of **massage strokes**

Keep your left hand on the right shoulder, slide your right hand under the back, so that your palm is facing up as it glides under the shoulder blade to clasp the shoulder muscles. Glide your hand down the back and when you get to the waist swivel your hand around to flow over the right hip and down the thigh, along the side of the calf, over the right foot and flowing onto the left knee, calf and foot in a continuous movement. It creates a wonderfully long smoothing stroke. Repeat as many times as you like, encouraging your partner to let go with every luxurious stroke. Help your partner unwind from the position gently before moving to the other side of the body, repositioning the support cushion on the other side, if needed, and reversing the twist.

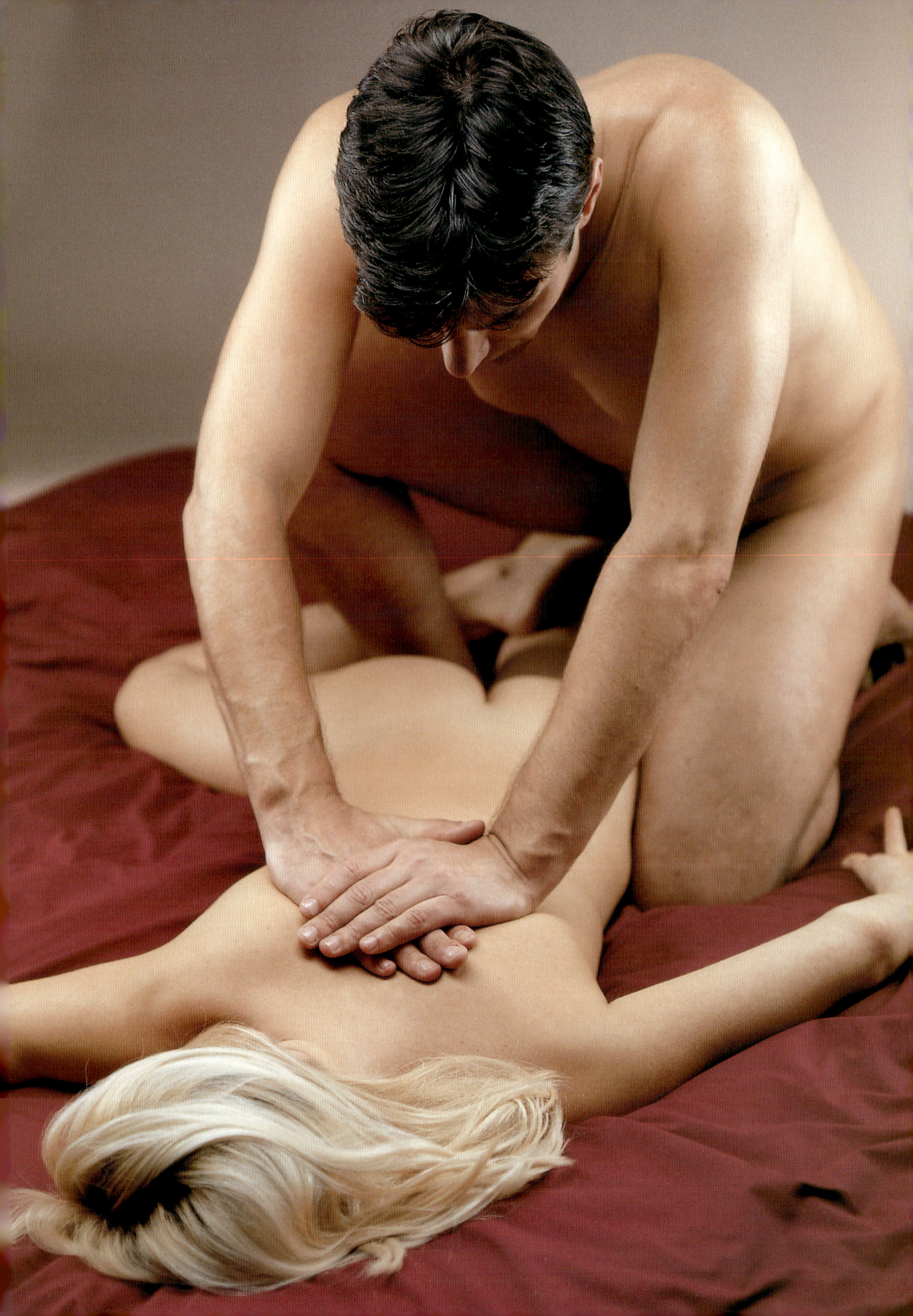

Spine: Kundalini balance

This massage sequence is a simple version of the balancing and cleansing routines used by the tantrics and yogis on the subtle energy centers of the body – the chakras or lotuses. Kundalini is the supreme energy that lies coiled at the very base of the spine. When it is awakened, it ascends through the body, awakening and recharging the vital and psychic bodies, illuminating the brain and leading to a heightened awareness.

Adopting a comfortable position

For this part of the massage, you partner will need to be lying on her front. At this stage of the massage it's perfectly acceptable for her to just turn over, with her head to one side, and collapse. However, not everyone is comfortable with the head stretched 90° to one side, as this position can constrict the airflow. One solution is to place a large cushion or pillow beneath the chest and allow the head to hang over it, thereby reducing the strain on the neck.

Alternatively, your partner may be more comfortable lying down in the following position, which also keeps the airways clear. From the cross-over position adopted in the Awakening Twist (see pages 106–107), either stand or lean over your partner and help her to roll the right shoulder and arm across the body to untwist the torso, and to pull the left arm and shoulder under the body. Take hold of your partner's right foot and position it on the back of the left knee. You can place a cushion beneath the right knee if it helps your partner to feel more comfortable.

Energy serpent

Once your partner is comfortably in position, kneel down with your left knee by her left hip. Step your right foot into the gap between the thighs. Flex your left foot and sit on your raised heel to create a secure seat for the first part of the sequence. With your favored or working hand, create a "V" shape between thumb and closed fingers, then place your supporting hand on top and entwine the thumbs to produce a bird's outline. In this position your hands can deliver pressure with control.

Start from muladhara (the root or base chakra at the coccyx or tailbone), and move your hands up the whole length of the spine to the sahasrara (the crown chakra situated on the top and center of the head), with clockwise circular movements. Hold on to the top of the head so that you can feel the heat and energy, until slowly releasing all pressure, allowing the powerful, free-flowing Kundalini energy serpent to ascend the whole length of the spine. Repeat this sequence as often as you wish, but always ascending the spine.

*allow the **powerful**, free-flowing Kundalini **energy serpent** to ascend the whole length of the spine*

Back: Snake charmer

In this sequence the massage giver emulates the pattern of a snake rising by making a swirling pattern with the hands that is synchronized with the rhythm and sway of the whole body – in other words, the masseur becomes the enigmatic moving snake. Stay in position, kneeling at your partner's thighs, for this part of the massage.

1 Place your hands on the top of one shoulder (the trapezius muscles) with the fingers spread and the thumbs touching. In a wavy snakelike motion, weave your hands to the left and the right, across the top of the shoulder on the other side and working slowly down the back to the small of the back.

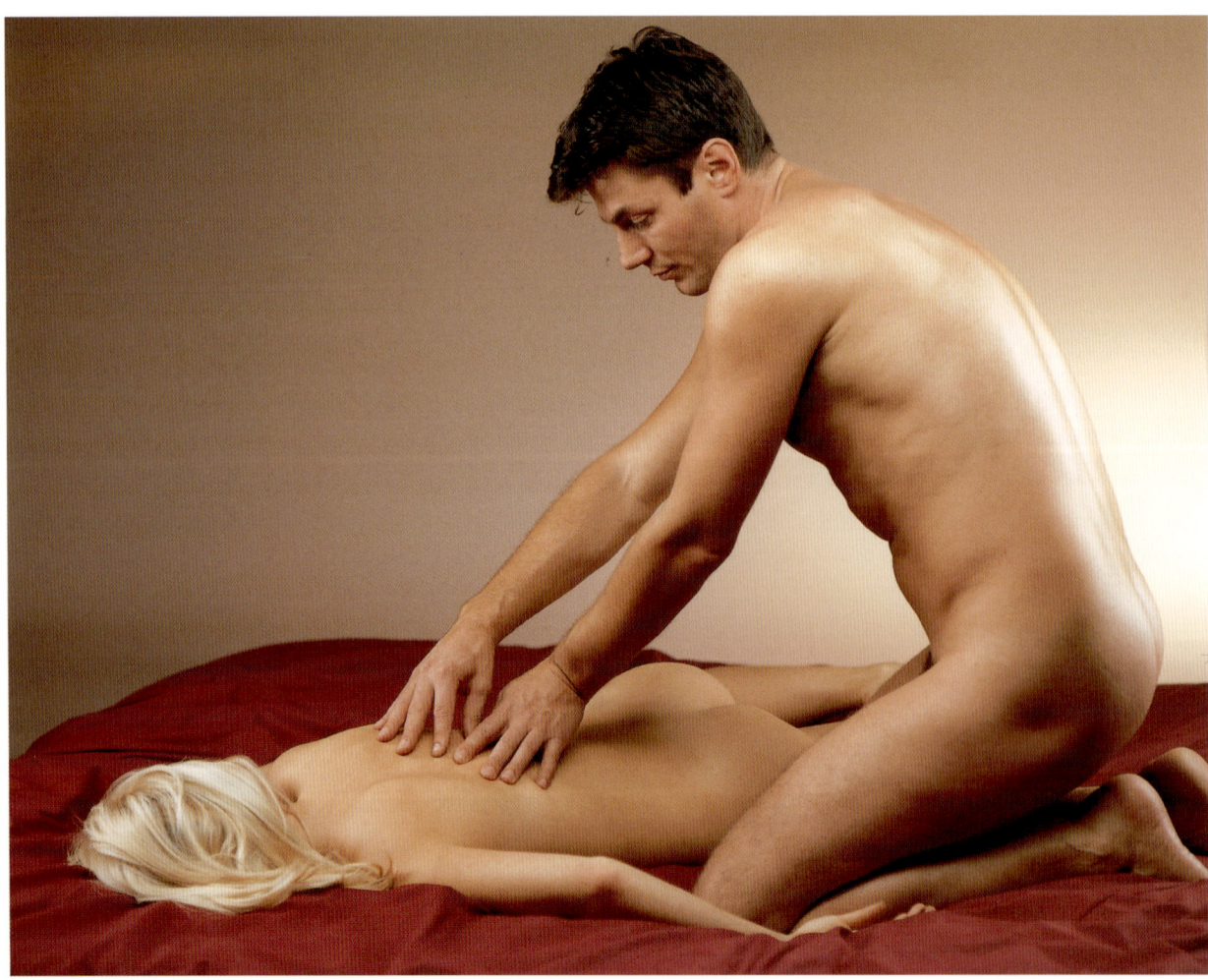

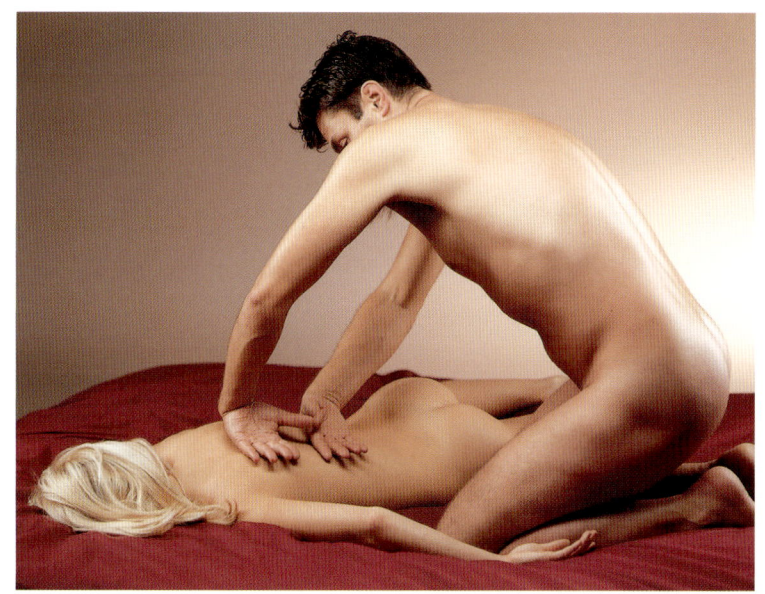

Flip the hands over, then stroke with the backs of the hands, weaving up the back in a serpentine stroke to the top of the spine. Then flip the hands once more and descend to the lumbar region again. Repeat a number of times to revitalize the spine.

As a finishing touch, interlace your fingers, one hand on top of the other, and make a large circuit of the whole of the back, working clockwise across the shoulders, down the right side of the back, across the pelvis and up the left side. Repeat as often as you wish.

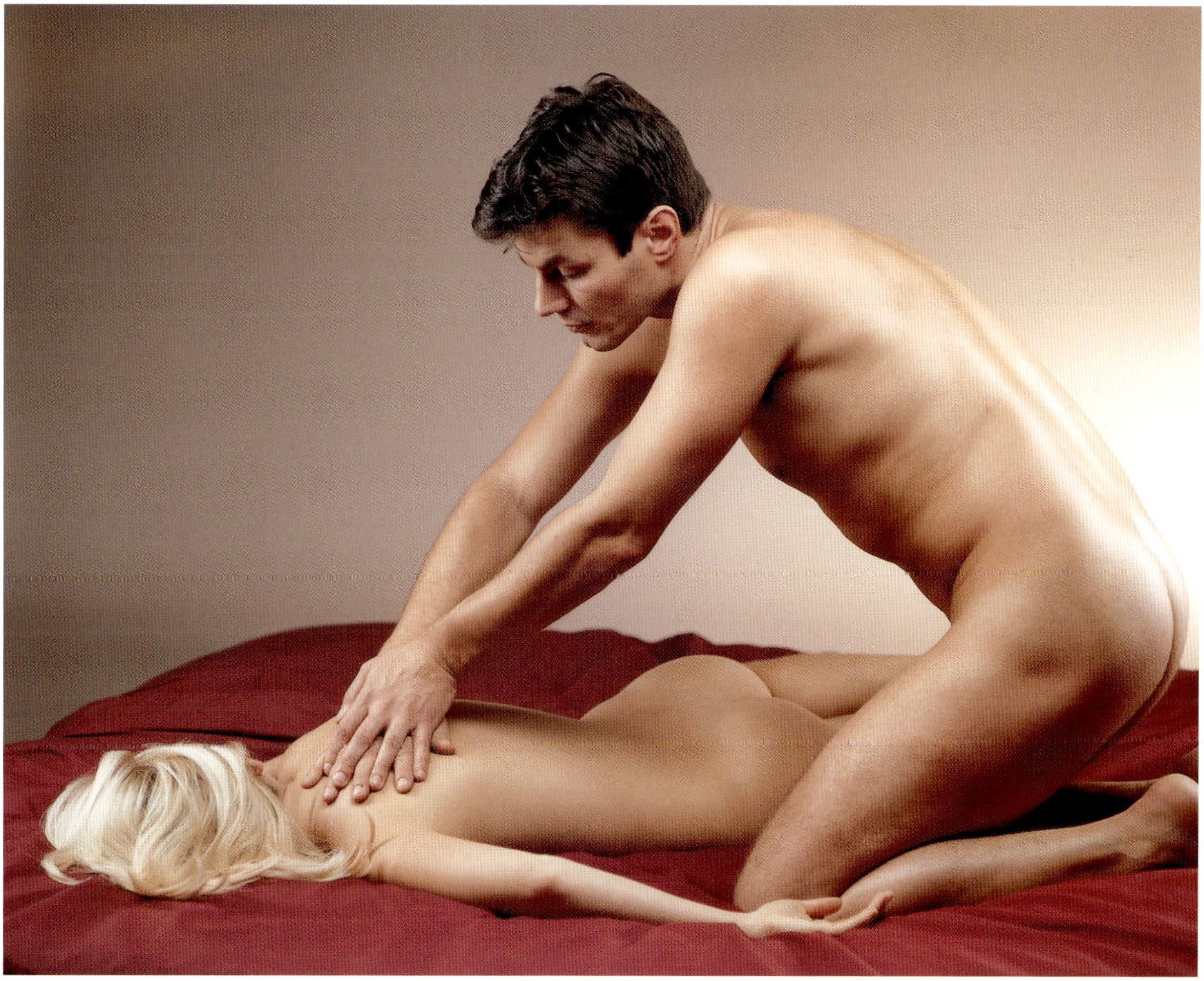

The buttocks and beyond

Ask your partner to relax fully on her front, supported by cushions and pillows. Having the buttocks raised in this way enhances the sense of vulnerability as the recipient cannot see or know what is going to happen, so be prepared for a range of reactions – from fearful to excited. If your partner doesn't feel safe or comfortable, simply use the circular buttock technique, smooth off and leave it at that.

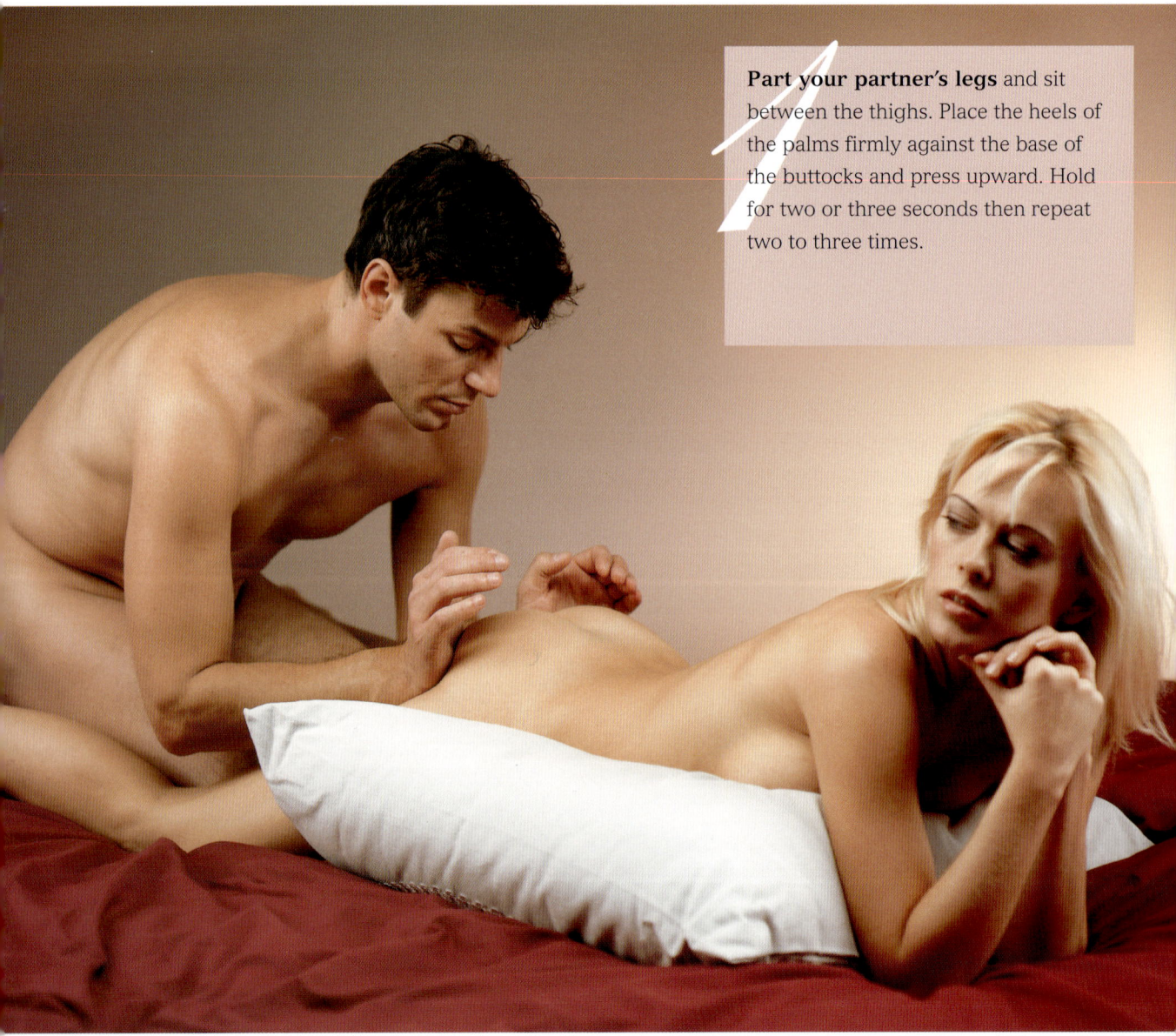

1 Part your partner's legs and sit between the thighs. Place the heels of the palms firmly against the base of the buttocks and press upward. Hold for two or three seconds then repeat two to three times.

Place both palms on the base of the buttocks. With fingers together, start to lightly massage the buttocks in two large outward circles. Slowly increase the pressure, giving a slight push against the base of the buttocks with the heel of the palms on each upward circuit.

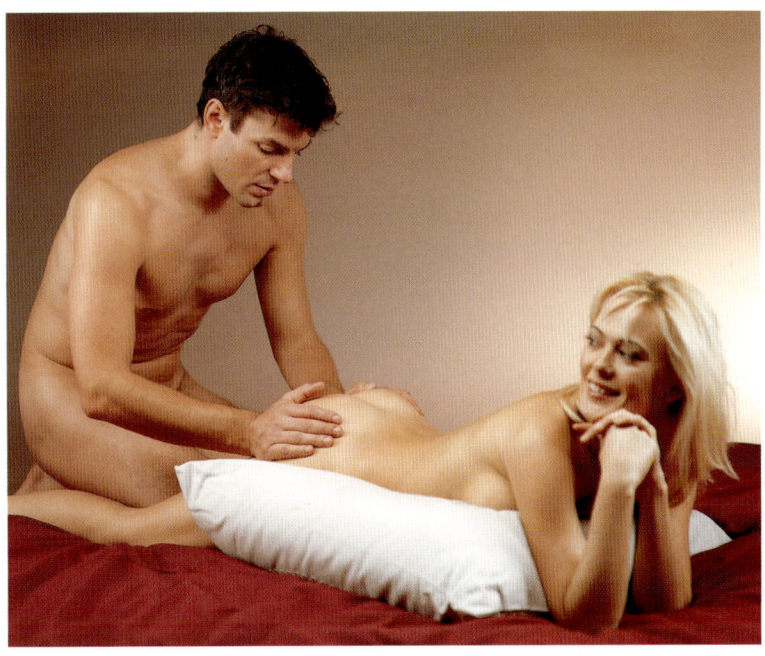

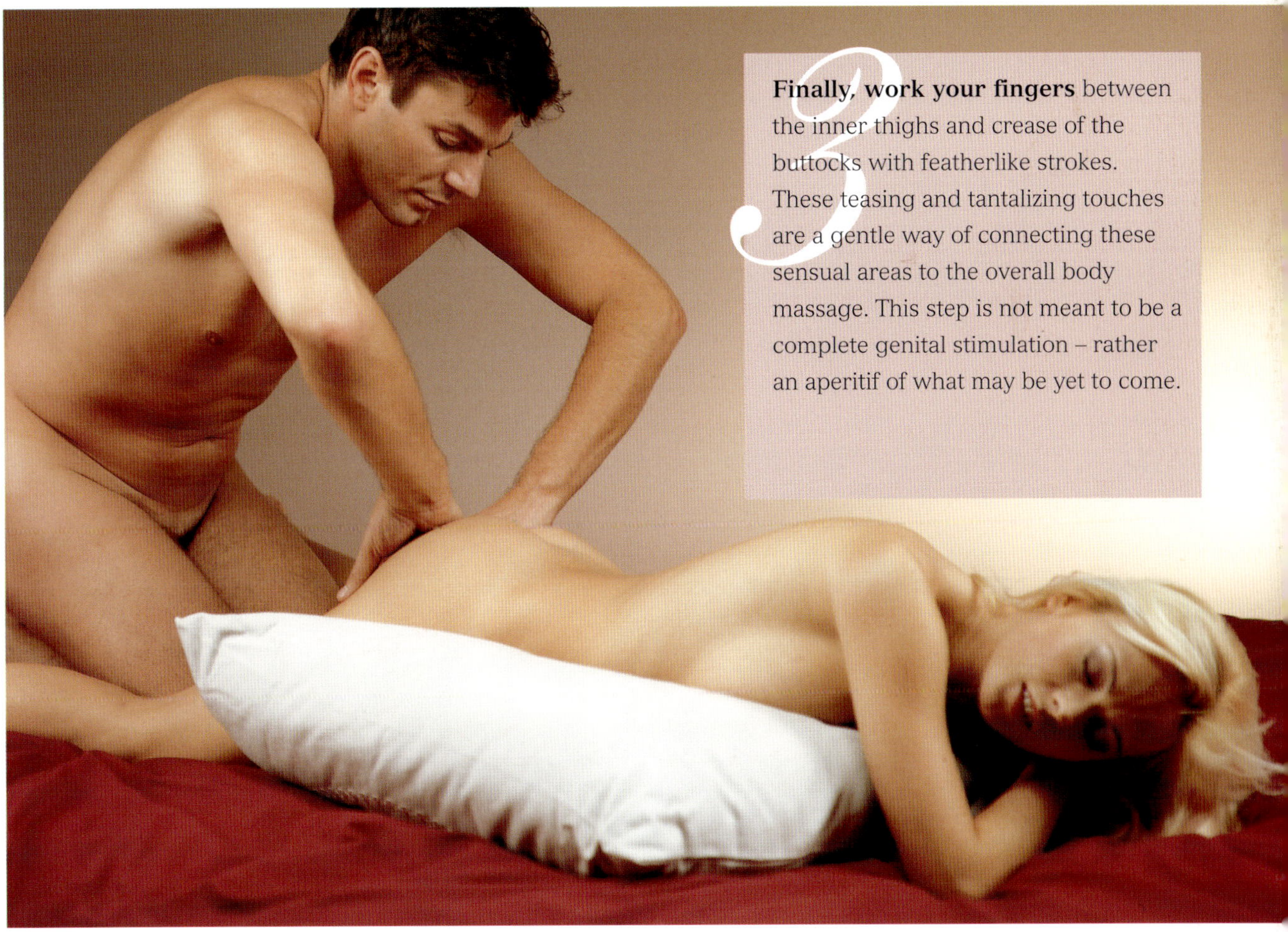

Finally, work your fingers between the inner thighs and crease of the buttocks with featherlike strokes. These teasing and tantalizing touches are a gentle way of connecting these sensual areas to the overall body massage. This step is not meant to be a complete genital stimulation – rather an aperitif of what may be yet to come.

Legs, calves and ankles

At this stage of the massage your partner's body is at a very good angle to work on. You use your own body as a prop, which is comforting for your partner. Move your sitting position backward to just below your partner's knee level. You can either sit or kneel with your knees apart so your thighs act as supports for your partner's shins. The techniques shown here act as draining, stretching and compressing agents that can help to increase circulation and relieve cramp and muscular tensions.

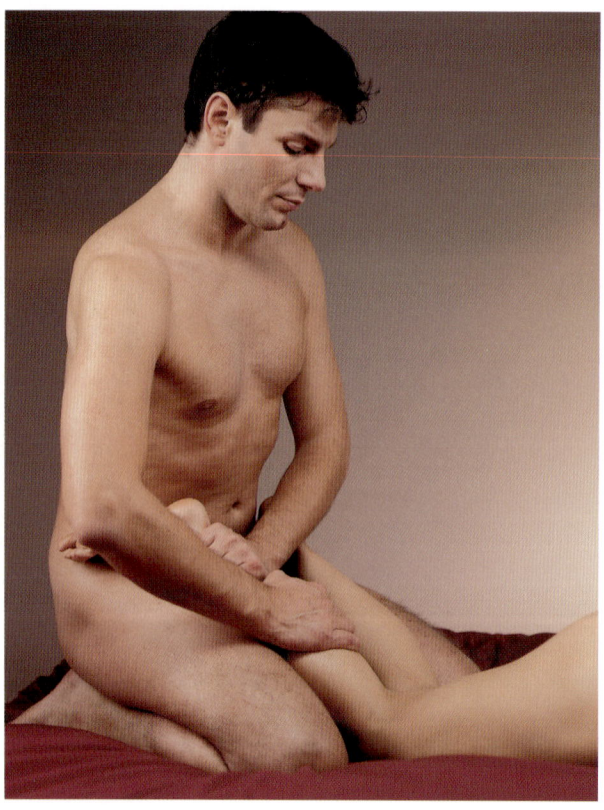

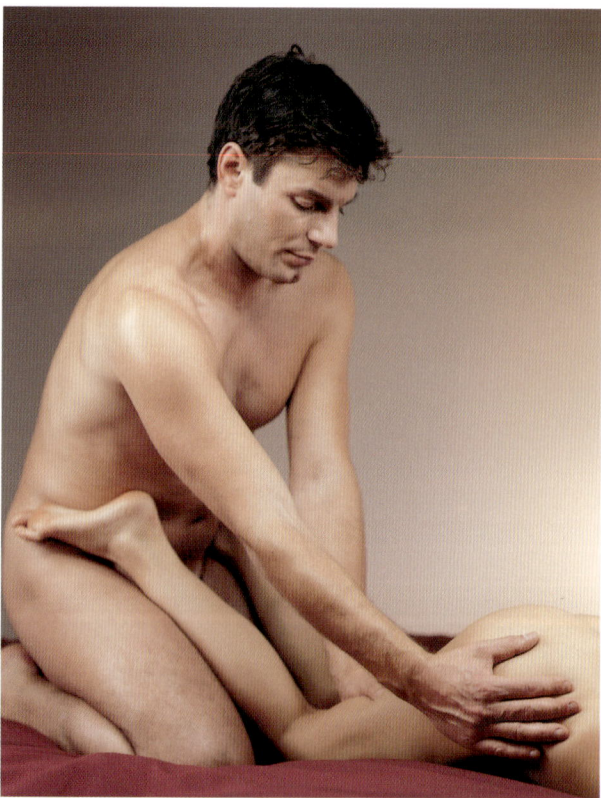

1 Lift your partner's legs and place them into the creases of your thighs and groin. Place the hands side by side on the lower calf of the right leg, just above the Achilles tendon, with the right hand closer to the knee. Then, molding the hands around the shape of the leg muscles, lean forward and push with your body weight, gliding both hands up the back of the calf, across the back of the knee and up the back of the thigh.

2 Now split the hands so the right hand caresses and smoothes around the shape of the buttock and hip while the left hand smoothes around the inner thigh. Repeat this move as often as you wish before moving on to the left leg.

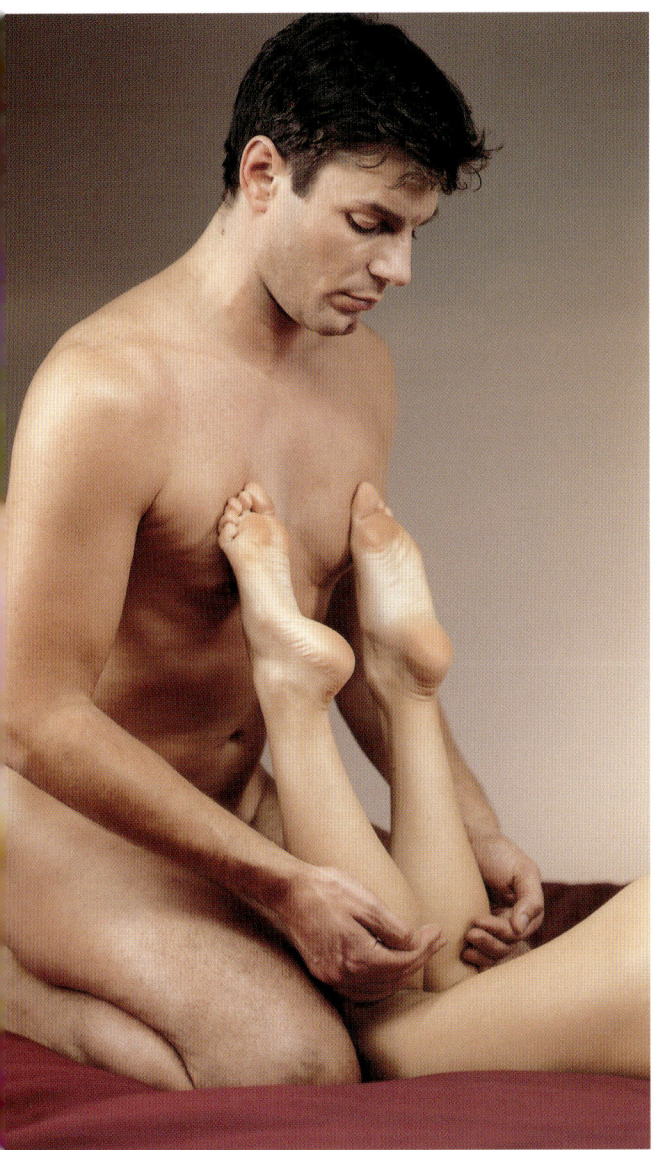 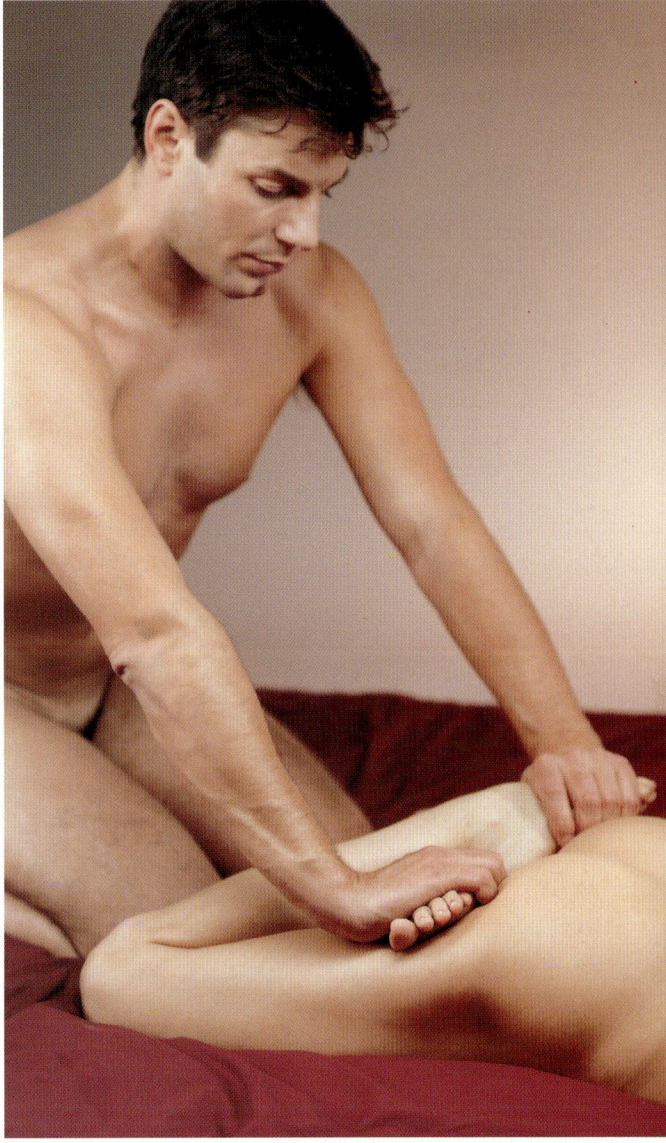

Clasp each ankle firmly with one hand with the edges of the hands and little fingers on the calf muscle just below the heel, then glide your hands down toward the backs of the knees in a smoothing stroke. Return the hands up the sides of the lower leg with a light touch then move them around to the front of the ankle, turning your hands over to create a "V" shape between thumb and index finger, then massaging down the shins to the front of the knee. Once again, return to the starting position by stroking up the sides of the legs. Establish a smoothing, caressing rhythm. Repeat as many times as you wish.

Separate your partner's knees as far as is comfortable. Cross the right ankle over the left and hold the toes. On your partner's out-breath, push the feet toward the buttocks, aiming to place the sole of each foot on the opposite buttock cheek, if possible. Take the movement slowly until you find the point of resistance and hold for two or three complete breaths. Then gently push a little further before releasing. Switch leg positions, with the left ankle over the right, and repeat the technique. This movement provides excellent relief for the lumbar back muscles and has a revitalizing effect on the energy meridians. Repeat the whole sequence, with both legs, two or three times.

Feet and toes

So many nerve endings and psychic energy points are located in the feet that even a little work on them can be worth a whole lot of massage elsewhere on the body. In addition, the ritual of foot washing epitomizes the ideal of loving service that will resonate in a range of cultures. Some people are extremely ticklish and will instinctively want to pull away from you unless you take charge and use firm and decisive techniques. Remember that the small bones of the feet are quite delicate, so don't be overzealous. That said, certain massage techniques are a case of being cruel to be kind.

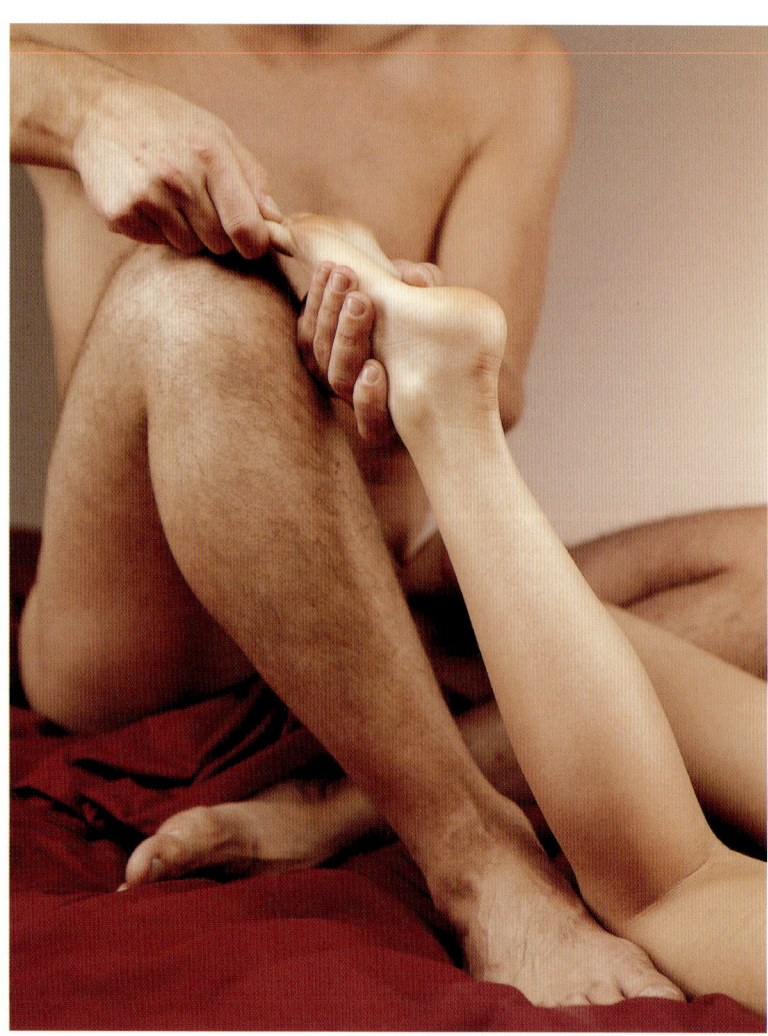

Toe-pulling Sitting square-on to your partner's feet and facing up the length of her body, bend your right leg and place your foot flat on the floor to create a "V" frame. Bend your left leg, push the knee out to the side and rest your partner's left leg on your left calf or thigh. Lift your partner's right leg and lay it along your right shin. Wrap your supporting hand around the top of the foot, with thumb resting on the instep, to keep the foot steady as you work. Place your working hand on the toes. Now pull and circle each toe in turn.

Hot tip

If you don't use oil, lotion or talc, (and, perhaps, even if you do!) you might care to use your teeth, tongue and lips instead of your hands in order to stimulate and lubricate the feet.

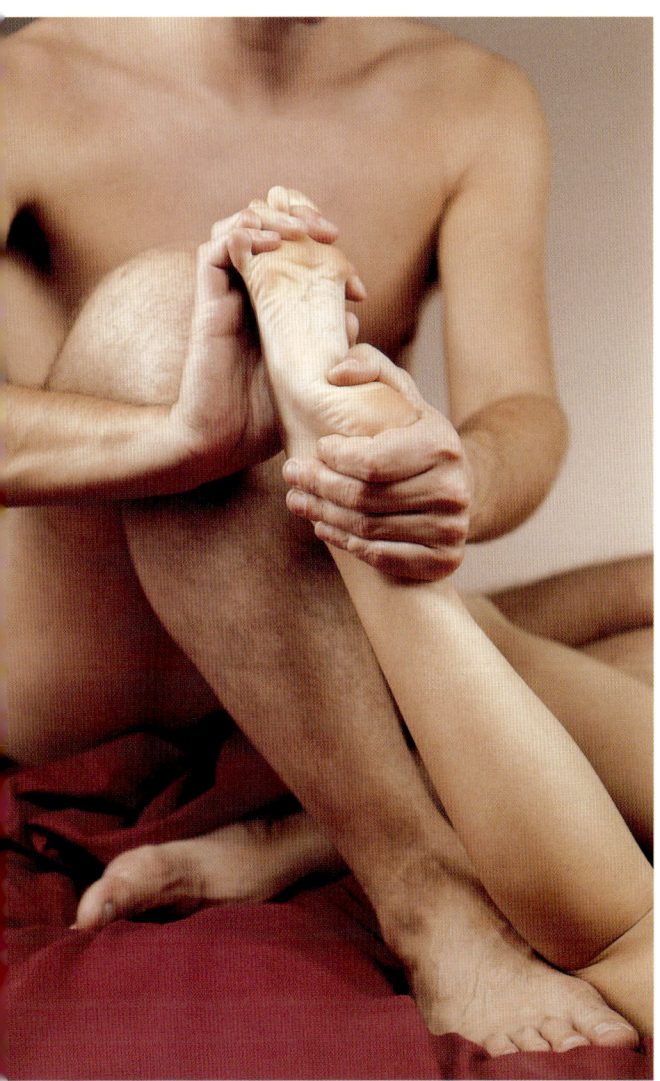 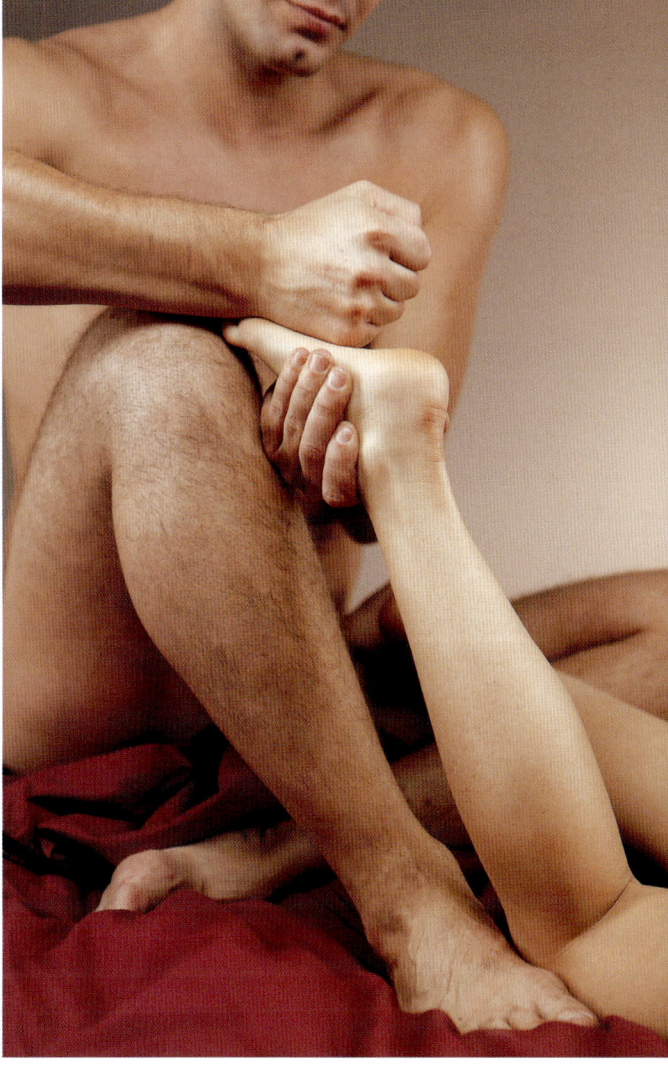

Spreading and twisting Interlace your fingers with your partner's toes. Flex the whole foot forward and backward slowly with a firm, consistent pressure. Repeat a few times then, firmly grasping the big toe in the left hand and the little toe in the right, push the right hand slowly but firmly away and pull the big toe, grasped in the left hand, toward you in a zig-zag stretch. Keeping hold of the big toe, "zig-zag" each toe in turn, using the big toe as the anchor point. Repeat two or three times as long as your partner is enjoying the experience. This technique creates a deliciously strong stretch in the metatarsal bones and will leave the whole foot revitalized and zinging with energy. Remember not to be too rushed or heavy handed. Listen to your partner for feedback.

Beating the rhythm Cradling the foot with the supporting left hand, use your right hand to execute a range of percussion techniques such as piano walking (see page 66), edging (see page 67), hacking (see page 74), pummeling (see page 75) and smacking (see page 77). As a finishing touch, sandwich the whole foot between your hands and gently pull off to the ends of the toes. Repeat two or three times. Now repeat steps 1 to 3 on the left foot. As a final touch, rest both of your partner's feet on your lap and cradle the insteps in your palms. Hold for a minute, then release.

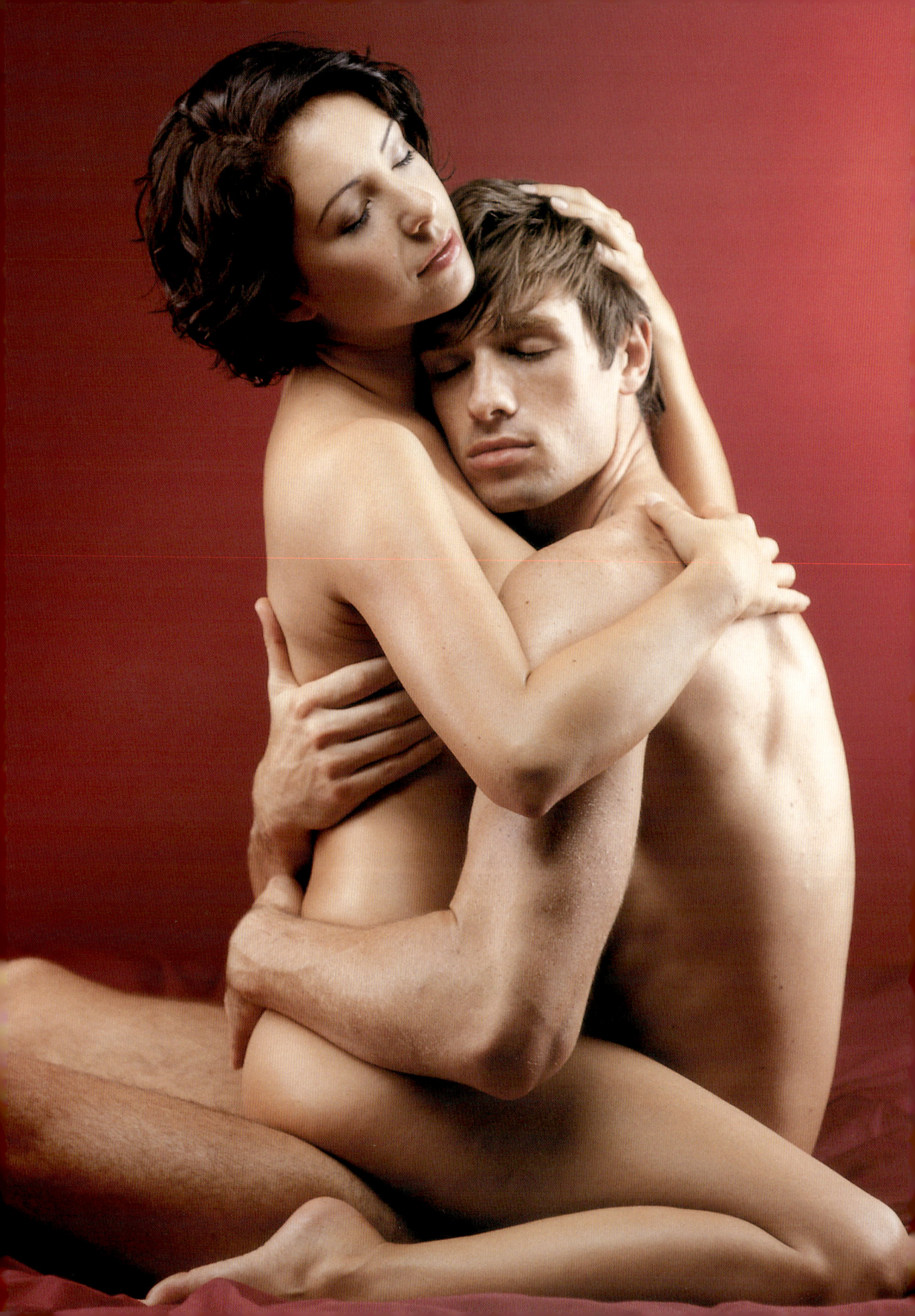

Afterglow

Calming and caressing techniques make bath time special as you unwind with bubbles and an essential scalp massage.

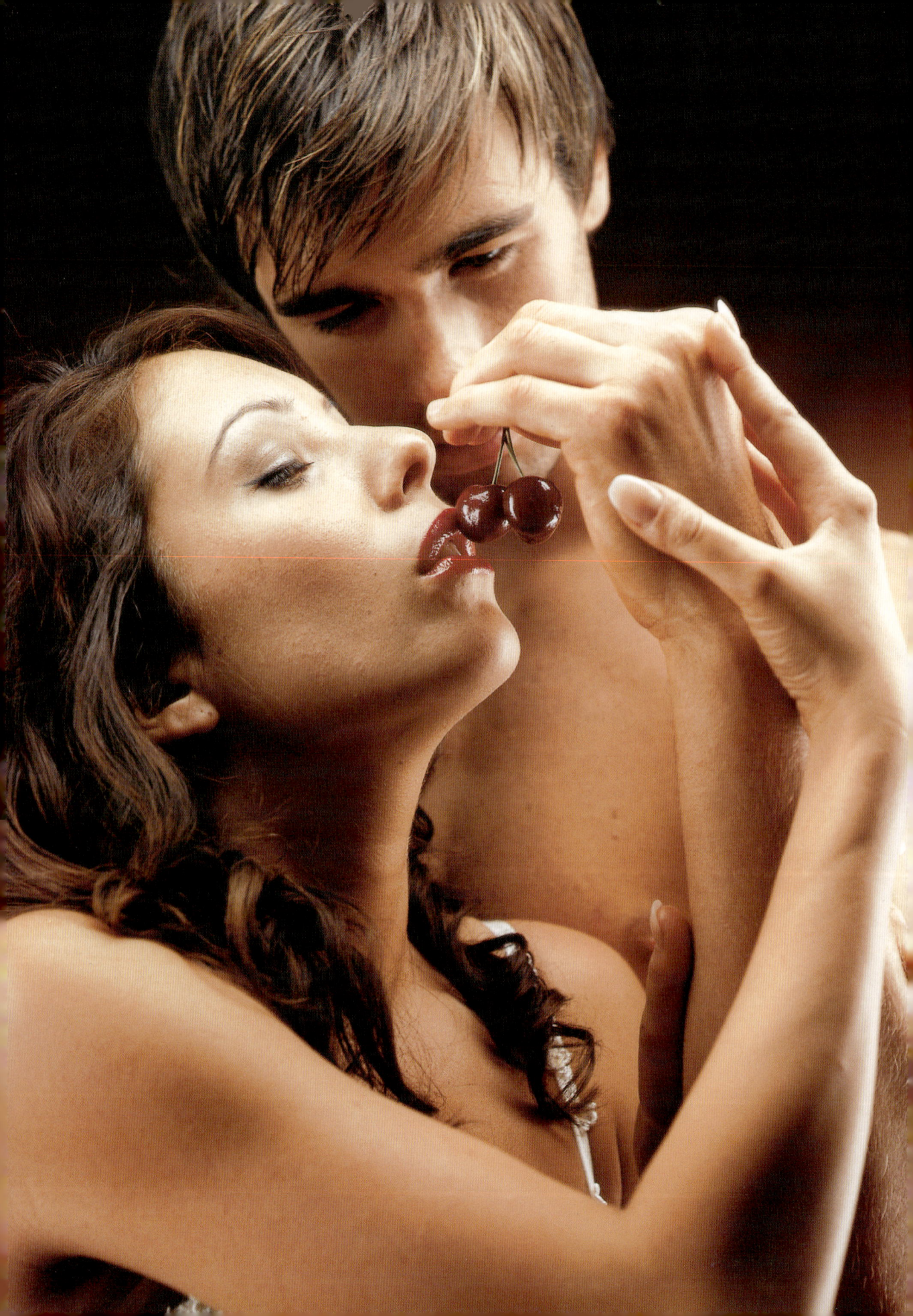

Bath-time seduction

A bath can be the perfect start or end to massage, and also to a wonderful sexual encounter, so why not create an erotic landscape in your bathroom? The trick to creating a powerful effect is to attract and delight all the senses – sight, sound, touch, taste and smell. Use your imagination to create the perfect mood for you and your partner – perhaps a tropical spa environment or a re-creation of a seductive fantasy.

Setting the scene

The cosy re-creation of a fantasy can be achieved with a few simple props. Light the bathroom with different shaped candles to create subdued – and flattering – lighting. Use mood music or CDs of natural sounds to create atmosphere. Preparation is all, so experiment with sound levels in advance. You can evoke a lush tropical environment with a few simple snatches of exotic birdsong and insect chorus, or a steamy night in New Orleans with some raunchy jazz.

Scented candles or incense can enhance the atmosphere, but if you plan to use essential aromatherapy oils in the bath itself you may not want a competing smell.

It is vital that the bathroom is warm and draft-free. Make sure there is plenty of hot water available. Ensure that there is an abundance of fluffy towels and robes on hand, and if you have a means of warming towels, such as a towel heater, perfect!

Forbidden fruit

If you intend to stay in the bath for any length of time you may like to prepare a plate of snacks. For a sense of luxury, choose rare or expensive items, those considered forbidden treats. If your theme is "jungle," go for tropical fruits such as passion fruit, pineapple, mangoes; for an Egyptian goddess or Roman seductress, use

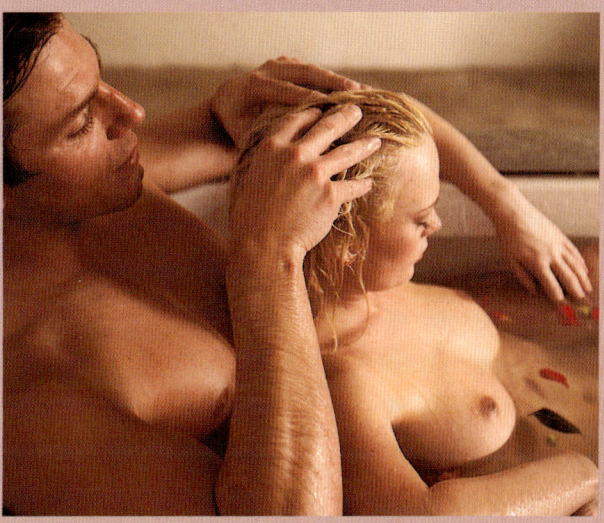

pomegranate, grapes, cherries and peaches; an *Arabian Nights* theme can be enhanced with a bite of figs, dates or Turkish Delight.

Flowers worn behind an ear, or flower petals sprinkled liberally in a bath are a link to the forces of the spiritual world, symbolizing a purge of our earthly impurities. Some flowers, such as rose, honeysuckle and jasmine, bring a more subtle aroma than any commercial product. A few fresh, aromatic herbs can add a spicy tang.

A bath-time session offers you the chance to demonstrate your creative talents and shows that you feel your partner is worth all the effort you have put into the creation – a powerful and erotic message to send to your beloved.

Anointing the head

This oil massage treatment is fast becoming a staple in the Orient. The benefits to hair conditioning and management are obvious. The sensuous delight of the technique is the delicious feeling of the warm oil poured on the forehead – a particularly sensitive area. The bathroom is probably the obvious choice of location, although by no means the only one. This should not be messy if you have a wide bowl to catch the flow of oil and are reasonably careful in your technique. It can be done on damp or dry hair and is particularly effective if combined with scalp massage.

Preparing the treatment

Firstly, warm approximately 8 ounces of pure, extra virgin, cold-pressed, olive oil. The very best quality is required for this technique to work as a tonic. Don't heat the oil quickly or to a very high temperature as this will destroy the oil's natural properties. It is vital that you test the temperature of the oil on the back of your partner's hand and obtain approval before application.

Your partner can be positioned leaning back in the bath for this treatment. Alternatively, she can lay on a raised massage surface with the neck supported by towels, or sit on a chair with the head tilted back slightly and, again, with the neck resting on towels. In both cases, place a large bowl on the floor to catch the flow of oil. This treatment is best performed in complete silence, with you and your partner listening to the sound of the flowing oil.

Going with the flow

Carefully and very slowly trickle, then pour the warm oil from a small pitcher onto a point a little above and between the eyebrows. This is traditionally recognized by some cultures as the site of the third eye and is the location of the vestigial pineal gland that opens up your inner world. The oil will flow over the brow, through the hair and onto the scalp. This is a blissful experience. The uniquely enjoyable aspect of the treatment is the sense of deep relaxation that is felt as the oil cascades over the head.

Whether your partner's hair is long or short, run your fingers through it to work the oil in, massaging the oil thoroughly into the scalp. With long hair, lightly squeeze off the surface oil by wringing it out in your hands.

Wrap a warm towel around your partner's head and allow her to rest for at least 30 minutes to enable the oils to penetrate the hair and scalp. Remove the towel and wash the hair in a mildly astringent shampoo of your choice. Rinse well, towel and allow the hair to dry naturally.

slowly trickle, then pour the warm oil... this is a blissful experience

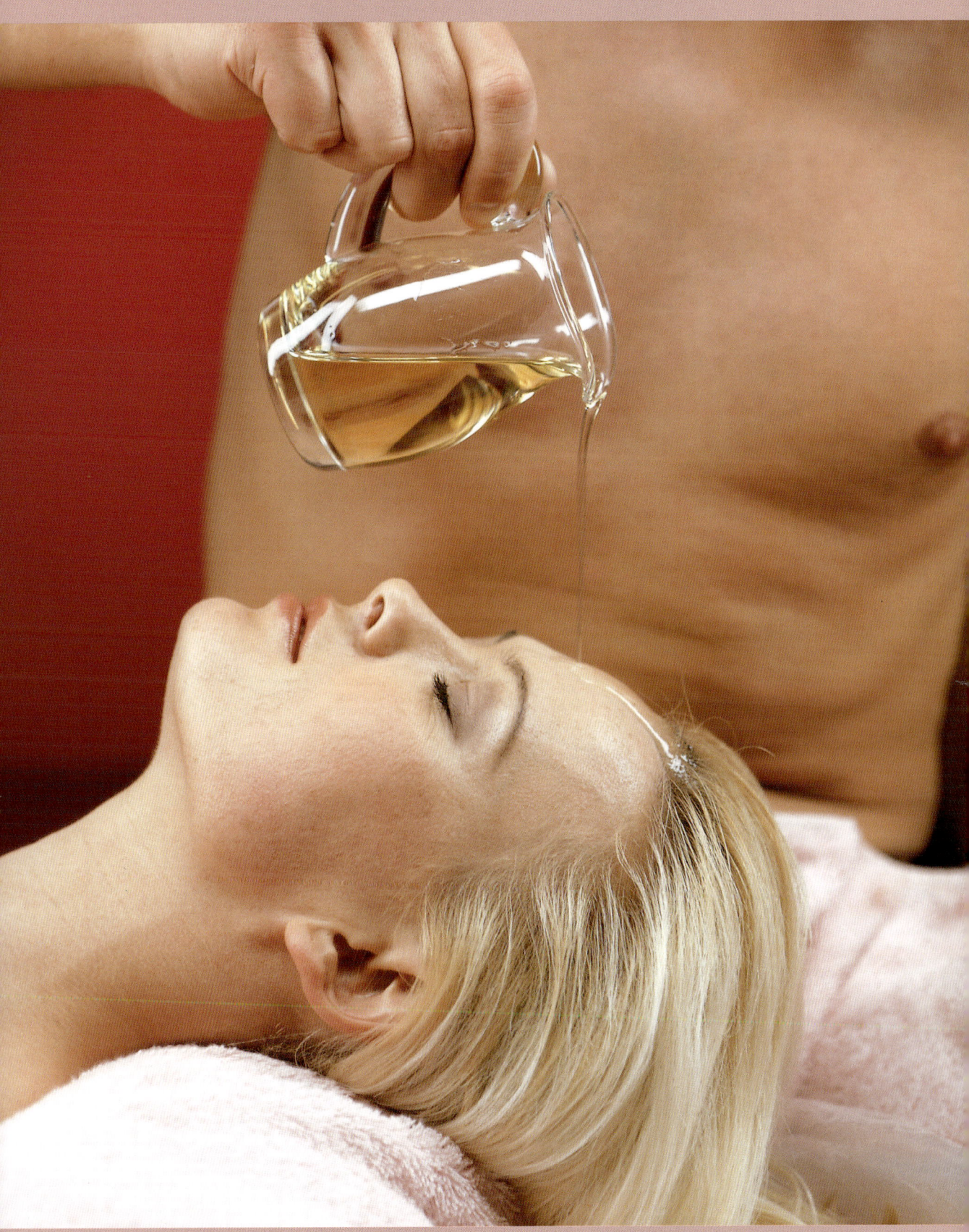

Anointing the head

Head and face

The following techniques are ideal bath-time or treats. They will invigorate and refresh your partner, preparing him for a passionate encounter, a relaxed evening or even a new work day. Why not create your own cleansing products? Consider using beaten egg yolks or avocado in place of hair conditioner and diluted lemon juice or vinegar as a light astringent tonic and rinsing aid.

Scalp massage

Using your partner's favorite shampoo, make a rich lather in his hair. Massage the whole of the scalp with small, circular movements of the fingertips. Work gradually outward with larger and larger circles to include the whole of the head. Rinse the shampoo off carefully, avoiding the eyes.

If your partner has very short hair, or none, you can still use the same scalp-moving techniques to great effect. Firmly plant your fingers variously behind the ears, above the temples and on your partner's forehead and, with a circular action, gently shift the whole layer across the skull to stimulate the circulation.

Hot tip

If you are washing one another's hair in the shower, change the water temperature from hot to cold, or vice versa, as a stimulant. Running your fingers through each other's hair and pulling the hair close to the scalp is a fantastic head tonic and can even relieve headaches and hangovers. After thoroughly drying one another, wrap a towel around your partner's head to form a turban. You could even give a gentle massage following the lines of the folds in the towel.

Traditional Thai replenishing facial

This famous Thai formula will leave the skin feeling plump and soft while helping to promote new cell growth. Three very simple ingredients will do the job: pure organic honey (which softens the skin), fresh lime juice (which peels the dead skin cells off the surface of the skin) and skinned and finely sliced cucumber (which hydrates the skin). After cleansing the face and neck with warm water, massage a mixture of two tablespoons of honey and eight drops of lime juice onto the face and neck and leave for ten minutes. Then cleanse the face with a warm, wet cloth and pat dry.

For the second part of the treatment, apply paper-thin slices of cucumber over the face and neck. The cucumber is a natural astringent that tightens the skin and replenishes moisture. Keep on for five to ten minutes while you and your partner are luxuriating in a bath, then remove. Wipe the face and neck and pat dry to finish.

invigorate and **refresh** your partner, **preparing** him for a **passionate** encounter

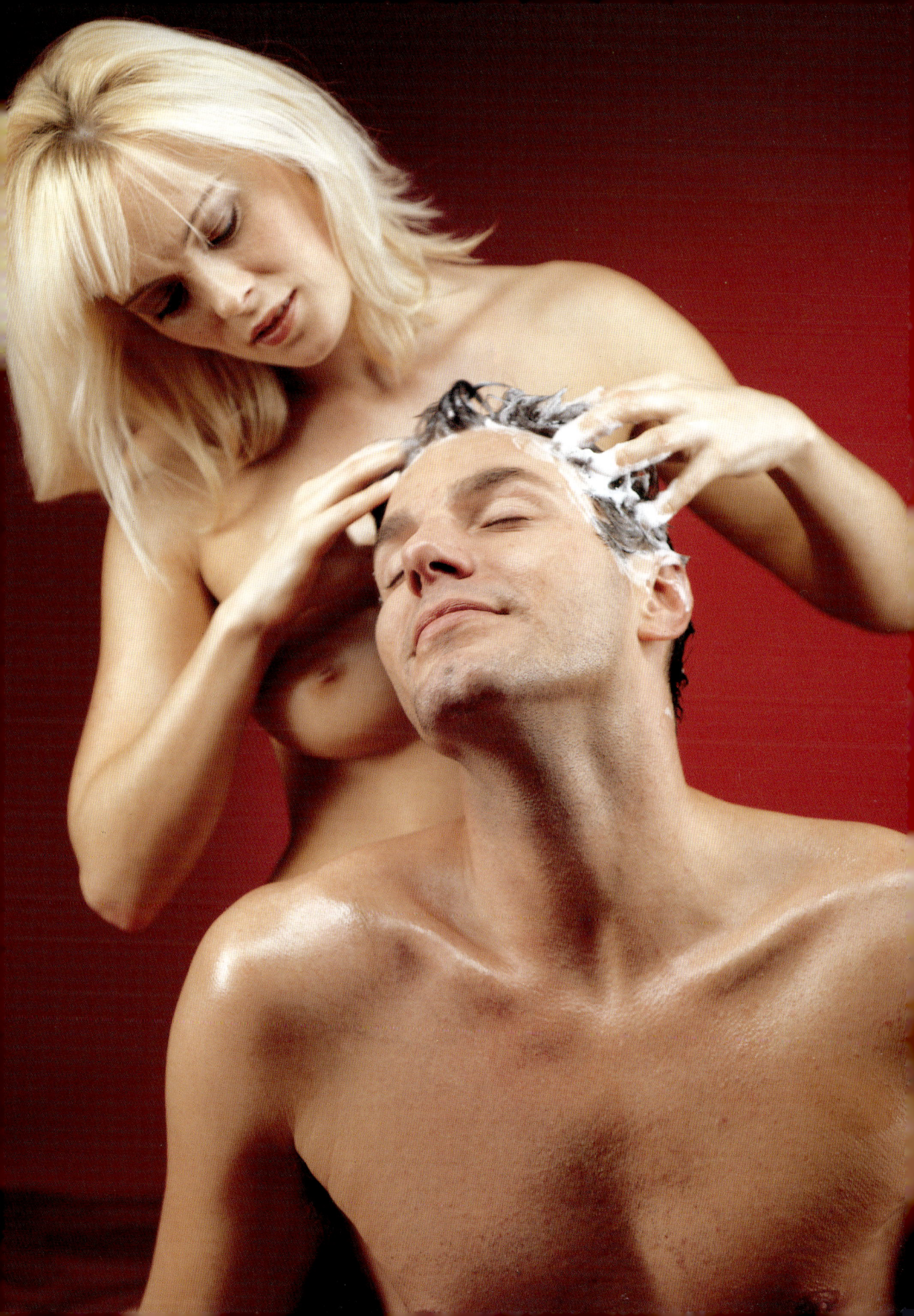

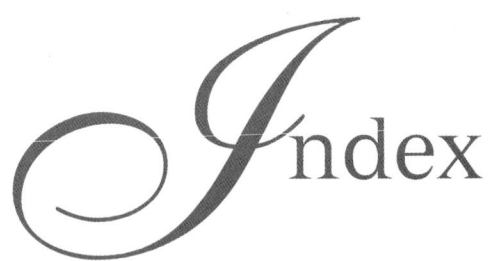

Index

A
ankles 115
arch friction 39
arms 98–99
aromatherapy 10, 21
assisted arch 90

B
back
  back-hand stroking 67
  lower back massage 42–43
  press 71, 88
  snake charmer 110–11
  warmer 84
bathing 120–21
blindfolding 55
body stretch 90
body wrap 91
breasts 30, 31
breathing, synchronized 12, 33
butterfly postures 86–7
buttocks 41, 44, 70–71, 77, 112–13

C D
calves 114
candles 10, 121
chakras 42, 109
chest 30–31
  expanding 78
chin pressing 94–95
chocolate 56–57
circular thumb pressure 72
clicking 76
coconut milk skin tonic 16
communication 6, 12
criss-crossing 65
cross-stretching 81
cupping 75
dress code 12

E
ears 27
edging 67
elbow press 71
environment 10
essential oils 10–11, 15, 18, 60, 100
  anointing the head 122–23
  and aromatherapy 21
exfoliation 16
eye contact 6, 10

F
face 26
  smoothing 94
  Thai replenishing facial 124
fan stroking 43
fantasy 12
feathers 48–49
feet 38–39, 116–17
  foot rocking 78
fir tree 62, 63
fire and ice 55
flowers 121
flying cobra 89
friction techniques 62–63
fruits 121

G
genitals 36–37, 55, 103
getting into the mood 12–13
getting started 10–11
gloves, silk 50–51

H I
hacking 74
hair
  play 52–53
  washing 124
head 94–95
  anointing 122–23
health issues 11
hip swaying 79
hot seat cobra 89
incense 10, 121
infinity ribbon 44–45

K L
kneading 38, 64–65
knuckling 39, 73
Kundalini Shakti (female serpent energy) 42
legs 40–41, 104–105, 114–15
lips 28
lotions 10, 21, 38, 100

M
making and breaking contact 10–11
massage surface 10
massage techniques 58–81
  before you begin 60–61
  beginning the massage 62–63
  body moves 78–79
  enlivening the skin 76–77
  getting deeper 64–65
  invigorating strokes 74–75
  smaller movements 72–73
  the spine 66–67
  stretches 80–81
  varying the sensations 68–69
  working the buttocks 70–71

muladhara chakra 42, 109
music 10, 121

N
neck
  massage 28–29
  neck and shoulder press 85
  neck and shoulders 96–97
nightwear 51
nipples 30, 31

P
palms 32–33
papaya body polish 16
penis 36, 37
piano walking 66
pleasure zones 24–45
  chest 30–31
  face, ears and scalp 26–27
  feet 38–39
  infinity ribbon 44–45
  inner thighs 36–37
  lower back 42–43
  palms and wrists 32–33
  stomach 34–35
  temples, lips and neck 28–29
  up to the buttocks 40–41
plucking 76
psychic shower 16
pulling 64
pulse 33
pummelling 75

R
racking 80
raking 68
restraints 55
role play 6, 12
rolling 69

S
"safe word" 12, 55
sahasrara (crown chakra) 109
scalp 27, 122, 124–25
scents 10, 22, 121
scratching 69
sex roles 6
shoulders 96–97
  shoulder rolling 85
showers 14–17
skin
  drying 18
  enlivening 76–77
  vibrant 16
smacking 77
spine 66–67
  avoiding the 10
  awakening twist 106–107
  Kundalini balance 108–109
spreading 63
squeezing 70
stomach 34–35
stretches 80–81
striking cobra 88
supported bridge 91
"supporting" hand 9
svadhisthana chakra 42

T
talcs 10, 11, 18, 100
Tantric sex 42
teasing and tantalizing 46–57
  chocolate 56–57
  feathers 48–49
  hair play 52–53
  silk gloves 50–51
  using playful touch 54–55
temples 28
Thai postures 82–91

  butterfly postures 86–87
  hot seat cobra 88–89
  statuesque stretches 90–91
  Thai bodywork 10, 84–85
therapy 12
thighs 36–37, 102–103
Three Heater meridian 33
thumb press 72
toes 116–17
top to toe 92–117
  arms 98–99
  awakening twist 106–107
  the buttocks and beyond
    112–13
  feet and toes 116–17
  head and face 94–95
  Kundalini balance 108–109
  legs, calves and ankles 114–15
  lower legs 104–105
  neck and shoulders 96–97
  snake charmer 110–11
  thighs and genitals 102–103
  torso 100–101
torso 100–101
towels 10, 18, 52, 121, 122, 124
trust 6
tying up partner 55

U V W Y
underwear, silk 51
vulva 36, 37, 103
warming up 62
"working" hand 9
wrists 33
Yoga bodywork 12

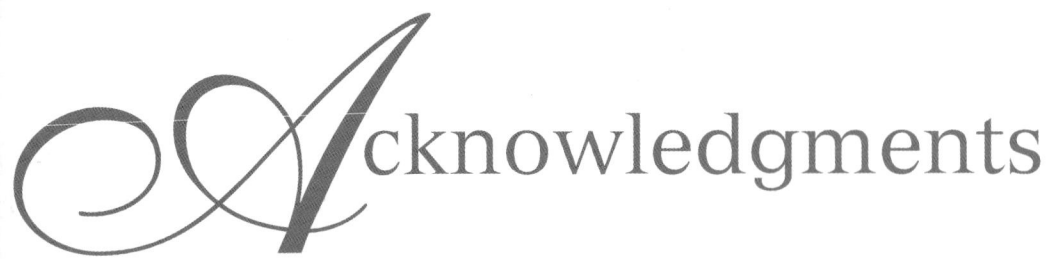

Acknowledgments

Authors' acknowledgments

As ever, all books are the result of many people's efforts and we all stand on the shoulders of our teachers. Firstly, we offer our respects and thanks to all those who, over the years, have taught us techniques or have been patient recipients of our burgeoning skills.

Regarding this book, our thanks go to those who helped with our own photographic pre-shoots: Julian, Jon, Bonnie, Arif, Natalie and Jude.

It is always a delight to work with true professionals. When helpful specialists combine solely to ensure the best possible results, ego has no place. Hamlyn has consistently provided friendly and talented staff, photographers, models, assistants and venues. We feel privileged to be in such company and the results surely speak for themselves.

In this regard our thanks go to Jane McIntosh, Executive Editor; Leanne Bryan, Editor; Tracy Killick, Creative Director; Karen Sawyer, Executive Art Editor; John Davis, Photographer; Dave Foster, Photographic Assistant; Stephen McIlmoyle, Make-up Artist; Janeanne Gilchrist, Photographer for the presentation; and Toko, Make-up Artist for the presentation. Thanks also to our wonderful models and to the staff at Big Sky Studios.

Rosalind Widdowson and Stephen Marriott

Publisher's acknowledgments

Executive Editor: Jane McIntosh
Editor: Leanne Bryan
Executive Art Editor: Karen Sawyer
Interior Design: Grade Design Consultants
Cover Design: what!design @ whatweb.com
Photographer: John Davis
Senior Production Controller: Manjit Sihra
Picture Library Manager: Jennifer Veall
U.S. Proofreader: Lee Micheaux

Picture acknowledgments

Special Photography: ©Octopus Publishing Group Limited/John Davis

Other photography: Octopus Publishing Group Limited/Janeanne Gilchrist 121